The Art of

C·h·a·n·g·e

Giorgio Nardone
Paul Watzlawick

Translated from the Italian by
Sally Davis and Michael Wyatt

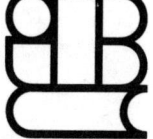

The Art of
C·h·a·n·g·e

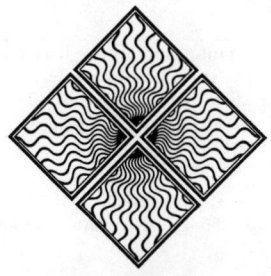

**Strategic Therapy and
Hypnotherapy Without Trance**

Jossey-Bass Publishers · San Francisco

This book was originally published as *L'Arte del cambiamento* © 1990 Gruppo Editoriale Fiorentino.

Substantial discounts on bulk quantities of Jossey-Bass books are available to corporations, professional associations, and other organizations. For details and discount information, contact the special sales department at Jossey-Bass Inc., Publishers. (415) 433-1740; Fax (415) 433-0499.

For sales outside the United States, contact Maxwell Macmillan International Publishing Group, 866 Third Avenue, New York, New York 10022.

Manufactured in the United States of America

The ink in this book is either soy- or vegetable-based and during the printing process emits fewer than half the volatile organic compounds (VOCs) emitted by petroleum-based ink.

Library of Congress Cataloging-in-Publication Data

Nardone, Giorgio.
    [L'Arte del cambiamento. English]
    The art of change : strategic therapy and hypnotherapy without trance / Giorgio Nardone, Paul Watzlawick ; translated from the Italian by Sally Davis and Michael Wyatt. — 1st ed.
    p.   cm. — (Jossey-Bass social and behavioral science series)
    Includes bibliographical references and index.
    ISBN 1-55542-499-6 (acid-free paper)
    1. Strategic therapy. 2. Hypnotism — Therapeutic use.
I. Watzlawick, Paul. II. Title. III. Series.
RC489.S76N3713   1993
616.85'20651 — dc20   92-32436
                                                           CIP

FIRST EDITION
HB Printing   10 9 8 7 6 5 4 3 2 1   *Code 9303*

The Jossey-Bass
Social and Behavioral
Science Series

Contents

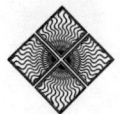

Preface

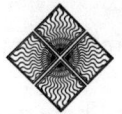

I take great pleasure in introducing a book that I consider to be an important contribution to the field of what is now known as strategic therapy or, more precisely, the practical application of systems theory and of the concept of self-organization to human problems.

Giorgio Nardone and I met years ago when I supervised part of his intensive training at the Brief Therapy Center in the Mental Research Institute (MRI) of Palo Alto, of which I am a member. Since then we have remained in contact, and I have thus been able to observe, and participate in, the establishment and growth of his Center for Strategic Therapy in Arezzo. Together we have organized a number of seminars and conferences in which we have presented the interactional (as opposed to the classical individual, retrospective, and analytical) view of problem formation and problem resolution to clinicians as well as to managers of large organizations.

The present book—whose Italian original *L'Arte del cambiamento* has found ready acceptance in my colleague's home country—gives a detailed account of Nardone's techniques and of the specific interventions that he has developed, especially in his work with clients suffering from anxiety, phobias, or obsessive-compulsive problems. It ends with a detailed survey and evaluation of the results obtained by these techniques. It is not, therefore, just a "cookbook" giving a superficial description of general guidelines, but rather a detailed account of both the theory and the application of this way of dealing with human problems.

The Strategic Therapy Approach

The considerable difference between the behavior of the therapist who employs strategic methods and that of the traditional psychotherapist can be made clearer by comparing the strategic approach to the game of chess. First, just as in a manual of chess, the rules of the game are given, together with the usual procedure from the first move to the checkmate. Subsequently, a series of effective moves and strategies are described. Finally, we are shown a few unusual games that illustrate how, by the interaction of moves and countermoves, the tactics of the game become extremely complex. The limitation of this analogy is that, unlike chess, therapy is not a zero-sum game, that is, a game in which there is always a winner and a loser. Rather, the game ends with both players (therapist and patient) sharing the win or the loss. By implication, then, any means used by strategic therapists in trying to win their and their patients' games take on a deep ethical value, even when they appear to be deliberately manipulative, because the aim is to find a rapid, effective solution to each patient's problems. When this is borne in mind, the accusation that traditional psychotherapists frequently make, that strategic therapists are treacherous manipulators, becomes devoid of meaning.

Overview of the Contents

Chapter One opens the book with my presentation of recent developments in the field of psychotherapy and goes on to define the theoretical and practical features that distinguish the strategic method from others.

Chapter Two offers an explanation of the basic conceptual characteristics of this method (hereafter referred to as "heresies," because they question the traditional "truths" of psychotherapy). They are the systemic, constructivist basis; a specific theory of persistence and change; and specific considerations regarding the formation and solution of human problems.

Chapter Three gives a detailed review of the historical developments of strategic therapy and emphasizes its Ericksonian, systemic nature. It also outlines some of the conceptual divergences contained in the formulations of the most important authors on strategic therapy.

The longest chapter, Chapter Four, deals with the techniques applied throughout the treatment, and also explains the main procedures (strategies) employed. This discourse does not consist merely of descriptions of the course of therapy and strategies but goes on to show their efficacy in altering people's behavior and opinions. Examples of research and experiments are included, as well as references to comparable problems encountered in other scientific contexts.

Chapter Five deals with actual cases of serious phobic and obsessive disorders and their specific treatment. The cases are presented systematically in a detailed four-stage format that shows the precise therapeutic aims of each one and the specific strategies used to achieve those aims. The cases demonstrate the efficacy of these methods and show how therapy can be a swift, well-planned journey whose point of departure, direction, destination, and length can be fairly clear from the beginning.

Chapter Six presents four interesting and unusual case histories. They demonstrate why, when seeking a solution to specific human problems, the therapist needs to combine a knowledge of systemic techniques with inventiveness and mental versatility. This is necessary because, occasionally, in order to find new, effective solutions to a problem, we must deviate from traditional conceptual schemes, from our usual ways of perceiving and reacting to our clients. Both knowledge and flexibility are essential for the rapid substitution of any ineffective solutions hitherto attempted.

Chapter Seven concludes the book on a note that is rare in our work: namely, a systematic, thorough evaluation of the results obtained by the application of this technique to a large and varied group of subjects over a two-year period. The outcomes prove that this approach is definitely efficacious: it can solve the problems to which it is applied, and results are obtained in a matter of weeks or months, as opposed to the years normally required by traditional psychotherapy.

Audience

I believe this book to be of fundamental importance for all professionals interested in psychotherapy based on systemic, Ericksonian concepts. I recommend it to all those who are interested in the formation and solution of human problems because, although essentially professional in nature, it is readable and comprehensible, and the strategies described may be applied not only to psychotherapy but also to more general, nonclinical interpersonal situations.

Palo Alto, California   Paul Watzlawick
November 1992

The Authors

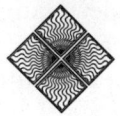

Giorgio Nardone is professor of brief psychotherapy at the Graduate School of Psychology, University of Siena, Italy. He is also director of the Center for Strategic Therapy in Arezzo and of the Italian Training Institute of Strategic Therapy, founded in 1989 in collaboration with the Mental Research Institute of Palo Alto, California. He obtained his Ph.D. degree (1987) in educational sciences from the University of Siena and also holds the title of specialist in psychology in the Department of Clinical Psychology of the School of Medicine, University of Siena. In 1985, 1986, 1987, and 1988 he trained for two months each in the systemic/strategic approach at the Mental Research Institute of Palo Alto.

Nardone's main research interests and activities lie in the theoretical study of the specific logical structures underlying human relations and in experimental, empirical, and clinical research into the effects of interpersonal communication in specific clinical cases. For several years he has also been engaged in the study of severe cases of anxiety, phobias, and panic attacks, and has published numerous articles on these subjects.

Paul Watzlawick has been a research associate at the Mental Research Institute of Palo Alto since 1960. He is also clinical professor emeritus at the Department of Psychiatry and Behavioral Sciences, Stanford University Medical Center; professor of communication sciences at the Centro Universitario Ticinese in Lugano, Switzerland; and guest lecturer at numerous universities and psychiatric training institutes in North and South America, Europe, and the Far East. Watzlawick received his Ph.D. degree (1949) in modern languages and philosophy from the University of Venice and his diploma in psychotherapy (1954) from the C. G. Jung Institute for Analytical Psychology in Zurich.

Watzlawick's present research interest lies in the practical application of systems theory and radical constructivism to human relationship systems, from marriages and families all the way to large organizations, corporations, and even international relations. He is author or coauthor of fourteen books that have been published in sixty-two foreign editions, and of more than a hundred book chapters or papers in professional journals. His books include *How Real is Real?* (1976), *The Invented Reality* (1984), and *Münchhausen's Pigtail, or: Psychotherapy and "Reality"* (1990). From 1957 to 1960 he was professor of abnormal psychology at the National University of El Salvador.

The Art of
C·h·a·n·g·e

If you would have a thing shrink,
You must first stretch it;
If you would have a thing weakened,
You must first strengthen it;
If you would have a thing laid aside,
You must first set it up;
If you would take from a thing,
You must first give to it.

—Lao Tzu, *Tao Te Ching*

Chapter 1

"If You Desire to See, Learn How to Act"

Paul Watzlawick

The title of this chapter is borrowed from an essay by the famous cybernetician Heinz von Foerster. He calls it his Aesthetic Imperative. Although postulated in a different context (Foerster, 1984), it nevertheless expresses what I consider an important aspect of the evolution of therapy. (The omission of the prefix *psycho-* before the word *therapy* is no slip, which I hope to be able to explain in the course of my presentation.) I do not know how exactly the inverse of von Foerster's Imperative — the idea that in order to *act* differently, one must first learn to *see* the world differently — arose and acquired dogmatic dominance in our field. For as different and even as contradictory as the classic schools and philosophies of psychotherapy are among themselves, one of the assumptions they firmly share is that the understanding of the origin and the evolution of a problem in the past is the precondition for its solution in the present. Undoubtedly, *one* compelling reason for this perspective is that it is embedded in the model of *linear* scientific thought and inquiry, a model that must be credited with the vertiginous progress of science during the last three hundred years.

Until the middle of the twentieth century, relatively few people questioned the supposedly final validity of a scientific worldview based on strictly deterministic, linear causality. Freud, for instance, saw no reason to doubt it. "At least in the older and more mature sciences, there is even today a solid ground-

Note: This chapter is reprinted, with minor emendations, from *The Evolution of Psychotherapy,* ed. Jeffrey K. Zeig (New York: Brunner/Mazel, 1987). Reprinted with permission from Brunner/Mazel and the Milton H. Erickson Foundation.

1

work which is only modified and improved, but no longer demolished" (Freud, 1964). This statement is of more than historic interest. Seen from the vantage point of the present time, it makes us aware of the evanescence of scientific paradigms — whether we have read Kuhn (1970) or not.

One would naively believe that the history of the twentieth century alone should leave no doubt about the horrifying consequences produced by the illusion of having found the ultimate truth and, therefore, the final solution. But the evolution of our field — since it usually is thirty years in arrears — has not quite arrived at this realization. Endless hours of "scientific" debates and tens of thousands of pages in books and scientific journals are still wasted in order to show that since "my way" of seeing reality is the right and true one, anybody who sees it differently is necessarily wrong. A good example of this fallacy is Edward Glover's book *Freud or Jung?* (1956), in which this eminent author employs approximately two hundred pages to say what could be said in one sentence, namely, that Jung was wrong because he did not agree with Freud. This, incidentally, is what Glover finally does himself on page 190 when he states, "As we have seen, the most consistent trend of Jungian psychology is its negation of every important aspect of Freudian theory." Clearly, to write such a book would have to be considered a waste of time, unless the author and his readers are convinced that their view is right and any other view *therefore* is wrong.

There is something else that our professional evolution no longer lets us disregard. The dogmatic assumption that the discovery of the real causes of the present problem constitute a *conditio sine qua non* (essential condition) for change creates what the philosopher Karl Popper has called a self-sealing proposition; that is, a hypothesis that is validated both by its success and its failure and thus becomes unfalsifiable. In practical terms, if a patient improves as a result of what in classical theory is called *insight,* this obviously proves the correctness of the hypothesis about the need to lift forgotten, repressed causes into consciousness. If the patient does not improve, this *proves* that the search for these causes has not yet proceeded deep enough into the past. The hypothesis wins either way.

A related consequence of the belief in possessing the ultimate truth is the ease with which the believer can dismiss any
evidence to the contrary. The mechanism involved here is well
known to philosophers of science, but usually not to clinicians.
A good example is the review of a book dealing with the behavior therapy of phobias. It culminates in the reviewer's statement that the author defines phobias "in a way that is acceptable
only to conditioning theorists and does not fulfil the criteria of
the psychiatric definition of this disorder. Therefore, his statements should not apply to phobias, but to some other condition" (Salzman, 1968, p. 476). The conclusion is inescapable:
a phobia that improves in response to behavior therapy is *for this
reason* no phobia. One gets the impression that it sometimes
seems more important to save the theory than the patient, and
one is reminded of Hegel's dictum: if the facts don't comply with
the theory, so much the worse for the facts. (Hegel was probably far too great a mind to have meant this in any other than
a facetious sense. But I may be wrong. Hegelian Marxism certainly means it dead seriously — and, again, the word *dead* is not
to be taken as a mere slip of the tongue.)

Finally, we can no longer afford to remain blind toward
yet another *epistemological error,* as Gregory Bateson might have
called it. Only too often we find that the limitations inherent
in a given *hypothesis* are attributed to the *phenomena* which that
hypothesis is supposed to elucidate. For instance, within the
framework of psychodynamic theory, symptom removal must
necessarily lead to symptom substitution and exacerbation —
not because this complication is in some sense inherent in the
nature of the human *mind,* but because it imposes itself logically and necessarily from the premises of that *theory.*

In the midst of such complicated thoughts, don't we all
occasionally have a disconcerting fantasy: if that little green man
from Mars arrived and asked us to explain our techniques for
affecting human change, and if we then told him, would he not
scratch his head (or its equivalent) in disbelief and ask us why
we have arrived at such complicated, abstruse, and farfetched
theories, rather than first of all investigating how human change
comes about naturally, spontaneously, and on an everyday basis? I, for one, would try to point out to him that there have

been at least some historic forerunners of that eminently reasonable and practical idea which Heinz von Foerster so well summarized in his Aesthetic Imperative. One of them is Franz Alexander, to whom we owe the important concept of the *corrective emotional experience*. He explains:

> It is not necessary — nor is it possible — during the course of treatment to recall *every* feeling that has been repressed. Therapeutic results can be achieved without the patient's recalling all important details of his past history; indeed, good therapeutic results have come in cases in which not a single forgotten memory has been brought to the surface. Ferenczi and Rank were among the first to recognize this principle and apply it to therapy. However, the early belief that the patient "suffers from memories" has so deeply penetrated the minds of the analysts that even today it is difficult for many to recognize that the patient is suffering not so much from his memories as from his incapacity to deal with his actual problems of the moment. The past events have of course prepared the way for his present difficulties, but then every person's reactions are dependent upon behavior patterns formed in the past [Alexander and French, 1946, p. 22].

And a little further on he states that "this new corrective experience may be supplied by the transference relationship, by new experiences in life, or by both" (p. 22). While Alexander attributes far greater importance to a patient's experiences in the transference situation (because these are not chance events, but are provided by the analyst's refusal to be forced into a parental role), he is quite aware also to what extent the outside world may provide just such random events as will effect profound and lasting change. In fact, in his *Psychoanalysis and Psychotherapy*, Alexander mentions specifically that "such intensive revelatory emotional experiences give us the clue for those puzzling therapeutic results which are obtained in a considerably shorter time than usual in psychoanalysis" (1956, p. 92). In this connection, Alexander (Alexander and French, 1946, pp. 68–70) refers to Victor Hugo's famous story of Jean Valjean in *Les Misérables*. Valjean is an imprisoned peasant who, upon his release from a long jail sentence that brutalized him even more, is caught stealing the bishopric's silver. He is brought before the bishop, but instead of calling him a thief, the bishop asks him very kindly why he left behind the two silver candlesticks that were also part of the bishop's gift to him. This kindness totally upsets Valjean's worldview. In the mental imbalance produced by the bishop's reframing of the situation, Valjean meets a little boy, Gervais, who is playing with his coins and drops a forty-sou piece. Valjean puts his foot on the coin and refuses to let Gervais have it back. The boy cries, desperately pleads for his money, and eventually runs away. Only then does it dawn on Valjean how hideously cruel his behavior — which only an hour earlier would have been a matter of course for him — now appears in light of the bishop's kindness toward him. He runs after Petit-Gervais but cannot find him.

Victor Hugo explains:

> He felt indistinctly that the priest's forgiveness was the most formidable assault by which he had been shaken; that his hardening would be permanent if he resisted this clemency; that if he yielded he must renounce that hatred with which the actions of other men had filled his soul during so many years, and which pleased him; that this time he must either conquer or be vanquished; and that the struggle, a colossal and final struggle, had begun between his wickedness and that man's goodness [Hugo, p. 95].

We must bear in mind that *Les Misérables* was written in 1862, half a century before the advent of psychoanalytic theory, and that it would be a bit preposterous to assume that the bishop was simply an early-day analyst. Rather, what Hugo shows is the timeless human experience of profound change arising out of an unexpected and unexpectable action by somebody.

I do not know whether another eminent psychiatrist and author, Michael Balint, has explicitly incorporated Franz Alexander's concept of the corrective emotional experience into his own work. However, in his book *The Basic Fault* (1968, pp. 128–129), he mentions the classic somersault incident, which provides an excellent illustration of such an experience. He was working with a patient, "an attractive, vivacious, rather flirtatious girl in her late twenties, whose main complaint was an inability to achieve anything." This was due, in part, to her "crippling fear of uncertainty whenever she had to take any risk, that is, take a decision." Balint describes how, after two years of psychoanalytic treatment,

> she was given the interpretation that apparently the most important thing for her was to keep her head safely up, with both feet firmly planted on the ground. In response, she mentioned that ever since her earliest childhood she could never do a somersault; although at various periods she tried desperately to do one. I then said: "What about it now?" — whereupon she got up from the couch and, to her great amazement, did a perfect somersault without any difficulty. This proved to be a real breakthrough. Many changes followed, in her emotional, social, and professional life, all towards greater freedom and elasticity. Moreover, she managed to get permission to sit for, and passed, a most difficult postgraduate professional examination, became engaged, and was married.

Balint then proceeds to use almost two pages to prove that this remarkable, immediate change was, after all, not in contradiction to object-relations theory. "I wish to emphasize," he concludes, "that *the satisfaction did not replace interpretation* [italics added], it was in addition to it" (p. 134).

The first comprehensive shift in the evolution of our understanding of human change occurred in 1937, when Jean Piaget published his seminal work, *La construction du réel chez l'enfant*, which became available in English in 1954 under the title *The Construction of Reality in the Child*. Here, Piaget proves on the basis of painstaking observations that the child literally *constructs* his reality by exploratory *actions*, rather than first forming an image of the world through his perceptions and *then* beginning to act accordingly. Only a few passages from his enormously detailed study can be quoted here to support this contention. In what Piaget calls the third stage of the development of object concepts, between three and six months of age, "the child begins to grasp what he sees, to bring before his eyes the objects he touches, in short to coordinate his visual universe with the tactile universe" (Piaget, 1954, p. 13). Later, in the same chapter, Piaget states that these actions lead to a greater degree of assumed object permanence (p. 41):

> A greater degree of permanence is attributed to vanished images, since the child expects to find them again not only in the very place where they were left but also in places within the extension of their trajectory (reaction to falling, interrupted prehension, etc.). But in comparing this stage with the following ones we prove that this permanence remains exclusively connected with the action in progress and does not yet imply the idea of substantial permanence independent of the organism's sphere of activity. All that the child assumes is that in continuing to turn his head or to lower it he will see a certain image which has just disappeared, that in lowering his hand he will again find the tactile impression experienced shortly before, etc.

And again, a little further on (pp. 42–43):

> In effect, at this stage the child does not know the mechanism of his own actions, and hence does not dissociate them from the things themselves; he knows only their total and indifferentiated schema (which we have called the schema of assimilation)

> comprising in a single act the data of external per-
> ception as well as the internal impressions that are
> effective and kinesthetic, etc., in nature. . . . The
> child's universe is still only a totality of pictures
> emerging from nothingness at the moment of the
> action, to return to nothingness at the moment
> when the action is finished. There is added to it only
> the circumstance that the images subsist no longer
> than before, because the child tries to make these
> actions last longer than in the past; in extending
> them either he rediscovers the vanished images or
> else he supposes them to be at his disposal in the
> very situation in which the act in progress began.

The importance of Piaget's findings for our work can hardly be
overrated. In the gradual unfolding of his research results, Piaget not only shows how the idea of a world "out there," indepen-
dent of oneself, is the outcome of exploratory *actions,* but also
explains the development of such basic concepts as causality,
time, and eventually, as he calls it, "the elaboration of the universe." If this be so, then, obviously, different actions may lead
to the construction of different "realities." However, before dis-
cussing this subject, some further milestones along the evolutionary path of therapy must be mentioned.

It may seem farfetched, indeed, that in order to reach the
next milestone I go back in time to Blaise Pascal, who, in his
Pensée 223, developed an argument that has become known as
Pascal's wager. It is of interest to us therapists because, although
theological in form, it deals with a problem very close to home.
Pascal examines the age-old question of how a nonbeliever can
arrive, by and through himself, at a state of faith. His suggestion is intriguing: *behave as if you already believed*—for instance, by
praying, using holy water, partaking in the sacraments, and so
forth. Out of these actions, faith will follow. And since there
is at least a probability that God exists, to say nothing of the
potential benefits (peace of mind and final salvation), your stakes
in this game are small. *"Qu'avez-vous à perdre* (What do you have
to lose)?" he asks rhetorically.

Pascal's wager gave rise to innumerable arguments, speculations, and treatises. Let me mention just one of them. In his fascinating book *Ulysses and the Sirens,* the Norwegian philosopher Jon Elster (1979, pp. 47–54) takes up Pascal's thought and goes on to show that one cannot decide to believe something without the necessity to *forget* the decision: "The implication of this argument is that the decision to believe can only be carried out successfully if accompanied by a decision to forget, viz., a decision to forget the decision to believe. This, however, is just as paradoxical as the decision to believe. . . . The most efficient procedure would be to start up a single causal process with the double effect of inducing belief *and* making you forget that it was ever started up. Asking to be hypnotized is one such mechanism" (p. 50). This seems crucial to my subject. To forget on purpose is one thing, and it is impossible. But to do something because the reason, impulse, or suggestion for this action comes from the outside, either as the result of a chance event or of a deliberate action or suggestion by someone else — in other words, in communicative interaction with another person — is quite another thing.

At this point I have to take up the evolution of modern family therapy, which no longer asks, *Why* is the identified patient behaving in this bizarre, irrational fashion? but rather, In what sort of human system does this behavior make sense and is it perhaps the only possible behavior? and, What sort of solutions has this system so far attempted? But these considerations would make my address mastodonic. Let me merely point out that at this juncture therapy has little, if anything, to do with concepts beginning with the prefix *psycho-,* such as psychology, psychopathology, psychotherapy. For it is no longer just the individual, monadic *psyche* that concerns us here, but the superindividual structures arising out of the interactions between individuals. Regrettably, it has to do with something that I wrote about years ago (Watzlawick, 1985), and repetitions are admittedly boring.

What I mean is that the vast majority of the problems we want to change are not problems related to the properties of objects or of situations — to the *reality of the first order,* as I have proposed to call it (Watzlawick, 1976, pp. 140–142) — but are related to the meaning, the sense, and the value that we have come to attribute to these objects or situations (their *second-order reality*). "It is not the things themselves that worry us, but the opinions that we have about those things," said Epictetus some 1,900 years ago. And most of us know the answer to the question about the difference between an optimist and a pessimist: the optimist says of a bottle of wine that it is half full; the pessimist says that it is half empty. The same reality of the first order — a bottle with some wine in it — but two very different second-order realities, resulting, in fact, in two different worlds. Seen in this way, one may say that all therapy is concerned with bringing about changes in the way people have constructed their second-order realities (which they are totally convinced are the *real* reality).

In traditional psychotherapy one attempts to achieve this through the use of *indicative* language, or description, explanation, confrontation, interpretation, and so forth. This is the language of classical science and of linear causality. However, it does not lend itself very well to the description of nonlinear, systemic phenomena (for example, human relationships); and it lends itself even less to the communication of new experiences and realizations for which the past provides no understanding and which lie outside a given person's reality construction.

But what other language is there? The answer is given, for instance, by George Spencer Brown (1973) in his book *Laws of Form,* where, almost as an aside, he defines the concept of *injunctive* language. Taking mathematical communication as his point of departure, he writes:

> It may be helpful at this stage to realize that the primary form of mathematical communication is not description, but injunction. In this respect it is comparable with practical art forms, like cookery, in which the taste of a cake, although literally indescribable, can be conveyed to a reader in the form of a set of injunctions called a recipe. Music is a similar art form. The composer does not even

> attempt to describe the set of sounds he has in mind,
> much less the set of feelings occasioned through
> them, but writes down a set of commands which,
> if they are obeyed by the reader, can result in a
> reproduction, to the reader, of the composer's origi-
> nal experience [p. 77].

And a little later (p. 78), he comments on the role of injunctive language in the training of scientists: "Even natural science appears to be more dependent upon injunction than we are usually prepared to admit. The professional initiation of the man of science consists not so much in reading the proper textbooks as in obeying injunctions such as 'look down that microscope.' But it is not out of order for men of science, having looked down the microscope, now to describe to each other, and to discuss amongst themselves, what they have seen, and to write papers and textbooks describing it."

In other words, if we manage to get clients to undertake actions that in and by themselves were always possible, but that the clients did not perform because in their second-order reality there was no sense or reason to carry them out, then through the very performance of these actions the clients will experience something that no amount of explaining and interpreting may ever have revealed or made attainable. And with this we have arrived at Heinz von Foerster's imperative: if you desire to see, learn how to act.

Needless to say, people may strenuously resist the request to perform such actions. The classical example is Galileo Galilei's contemporaries who disdained to look through his telescope because they *knew* without looking that what he claimed to see *could not* be the case (within the limits of their second-order reality, that is, geocentricity). Remember—if the facts don't comply with the theory, so much the worse for the facts.

To anybody acquainted with Milton Erickson's work, the concept of injunctive language, if not the designation, is nothing new. In the second half of his professional life, Erickson increasingly utilized direct behavior prescriptions outside trance states in order to achieve therapeutic change. Being a master in dealing with resistance, he gave us an important rule: learn and use the patient's language. This, too, is a radical departure from classical psychotherapy, where a great deal of time is spent in the beginning stages of treatment in the attempt to teach the patient a new "language," that is, the conceptualizations of the particular school of therapy that the therapist subscribes to. Only when patients have begun to think in terms of this epistemology, to see themselves, their problems, their lives, in this perspective, is therapeutic change attempted within this framework. Needless to say, this process may take a long time. In hypnotherapy the opposite takes place; it is the therapist who learns the patient's language and reality construction (as we would call it nowadays), and then gives suggestions in this language, thereby minimizing resistance (and time).

Outside its therapeutic applications, the study of injunctive language had its origins in the work of the Austrian philosopher Ernst Mally. In his book *Grundgesetze des Sollens* (1926), Mally developed a theory of wishes and commands that he called *deontic* logic.

Another important contribution to this subject can be found in the work of British philosopher of language John L. Austin (1962). In his famous Harvard Lectures (in 1955), he identified a particular form of communication which he called *performative speech acts* or *performative sentences.* "The term *performative* will be used in a variety of cognate ways and constructions, much as the term *imperative* is. The name is derived, of course, from *perform,* the usual verb with the noun *action:* it indicates that the issuing of the utterance is the performing of an action — it is not normally thought of as just saying something" (p. 6).

For instance, if I say, "He promises to return the book tomorrow," I describe (in indicative language) an action, a speech act, by that person. But if I say, "I promise to return the book tomorrow," saying "I promise" *is itself* the promise, the action. In Austin's terminology, the first example (the description) is called a *constative,* while the second is a *performative* speech act. In Lecture IV, Austin points to the difference between the statements "I am running" and "I apologize." The former is a mere report of an action; the latter is *itself* the action, *is* the apology.

Other examples from everyday life are "I take this woman to be my lawful wedded wife," "I name this ship *Queen Elizabeth*," "I give and bequeath my watch to my brother."

In all of these and in countless analogous speech acts, a concrete result is achieved, while my saying "winter is coming" does not make the winter come. Of course, a number of preconditions have to be met for a performative speech act to obtain or be effective. For instance, past disappointment or lies may make me doubt the promise; the apology must not be offered in a sneering, sarcastic tone of voice; the ceremony of naming a ship has to be an established procedure in a given culture. But if and when these preconditions are met, a reality is literally created by the performative utterance, and whoever subsequently referred to that ship as the *Joseph Stalin* would be considered somewhat deranged.

With these remarks I have barely scratched the surface of Austin's work in this specialized area of linguistics, that is, his ideas on "how to do things with words." But I hope that even these brief references will reveal some of the richness and the relevance of it for our work.

Of a particularly mind-boggling effect are the so-called self-fulfilling prophecies, known to unorthodox therapists and stockbrokers alike—but not to weather forecasters: imagined effect produces concrete cause; the future (not the past) determines the present; the prophecy of the event leads to the event of the prophecy (Watzlawick, 1984).

I am convinced that injunctive language will acquire a central place within the frame of modern therapeutic techniques. Of course, it has always occupied this place in hypnotherapy. For what is a hypnotic suggestion if not an injunction to behave *as if* something were the case—something which does become the case (that is, becomes "real") as a result of having been carried out. But this is tantamount to saying that injunctions can literally *construct* realities, just as chance events can have this effect not only in human lives, but are known to have it in cosmic as well as biological evolution. In this connection, it would be tempting to go off on a tangent, into questions of self-organization, or what Prigogine (1980) called *dissipative structures*—a subject that would exceed the limits of my competence and my time.

But, why is there a crucial difference between something originating within myself and an impulse that comes from the outside? Several answers offer themselves, but none seems convincing. That it is so is no secret. In our own lives we have little difficulty creating the same disaster as our so-called patients do in their lives, and to tickle oneself is never as ticklish as being tickled by somebody else.

However, to go back to Pascal. There are two little words in his behavior prescription that merit attention: behave *as if* you already believed. They clearly point to the initially quite fictional nature of this class of interventions. And it is this fictionality that creates doubts. The common objection is that even if they are successful, their effect cannot last. After all, they are only make-believe, an as-if fiction. Sooner or later, probably sooner, they must run up against the hard facts of reality and be defeated.

Here is the counterargument: The idea of introducing an as-if assumption into a situation and thereby arriving at concrete results is by no means a recent one. It goes back at least to the year 1911, when the German philosopher Hans Vaihinger published his *Philosophie des Als Ob,* whose English title is *The Philosophy of "As If"* (1924). If it were not for the fact that Alfred Adler (and, to a lesser degree, also Freud) had already recognized the importance of these ideas, their application to our field could very well be called the Therapy of As If, or the therapy of "planned chance events."

Again, I do not see how I can avoid repeating here something that I mentioned years ago: what Vaihinger presents in a mere eight hundred pages is an astounding richness of examples, drawn from all branches of science as well as from everyday life, showing that we *always* work with unproven and unprovable assumptions which, nevertheless, lead to concrete, practical results. There is not and there never will be any proof that man is really endowed with free will and is therefore responsible for his actions. However, I know of no society, culture, or civilization, past or present, in which people did not behave *as if* this were the case, because without this fictitious assumption, practical, concrete social order would be impossible. The idea of the square root of minus one is totally fictional. It is not only intellectually unimaginable, it also violates the basic rules of arithmetic; yet, mathematicians, physicists, engineers, computer programmers, and others have nonchalantly included this fiction in their equations and have arrived at very concrete results—such as modern electronics.

The rules and patterns of interaction that a family or systems therapist believes to observe are quite obviously *read* into the observed phenomena by the therapist. They are not really there. And yet, to conduct therapy *as if* these patterns existed can lead to practical and quick results. Thus, the question is no longer, Which school of therapy is *right*? but rather, Which as-if assumptions produce better concrete results? Maybe the decline of dogma is approaching.

Maybe not. However, what can be said—by way of an outlook on the evolution of our field—is that this way of conceptualizing and of trying to resolve human problems is gaining increasing attention as the traditional techniques of problem resolution seem to be reaching the limits of their usefulness. We are beginning to apply these methods to what may be called the specific pathologies of large systems. It does not seem totally utopian to imagine their application even to some of the most pressing and threatening problems of our planet, such as the maintenance of peace or the preservation of our biosphere. However, these attempts are too often beset by the same basic mistake that plays havoc in clinical work, namely, the assumption that since the problems are of enormous proportion, only some equally enormous, transcending solution has any chance of succeeding.

The opposite appears to be the case. If we look at the history of the last few centuries, beginning with the French Revolution or even with the Inquisition, we see that invariably and without exception the worst atrocities were the direct result of grandiose and utopian attempts at improving the world. What the philosopher Karl Popper calls "a policy of small steps" is unacceptable to idealists and ideologists. Remember the aphorism that Gregory Bateson often mentioned: "He who would do good must do so in minute particulars. The general good is the plea of patriots, politicians, and knaves."

To convince ourselves, we only have to look at nature. Great changes are always catastrophic and cataclysmic. Negentropy—or *anotropy,* as my friend George Vassiliou in Athens prefers to call it, in order to avoid the double negative—works patiently, silently, in small steps; yet it is the force behind evolution, self-organization, and higher complexity in the universe. I think that if we, as therapists, begin to see ourselves as the servants of negentropy, we will fulfill our function better than we do as supposed world-improvers and gurus. Heinz von Foerster (1984) defined this function in his Ethical Imperative: act always so as to increase the number of choices.

Many centuries ago this same outlook was expressed in a charming story: After his death, the Sufi Abu Bakr Shibli appeared to one of his friends in a dream. "How has God treated you?" the friend asked. And the Sufi answered, "As I stood before His throne, He asked me, 'Do you know why I am forgiving you?' And I said, 'Because of my good deeds?' And God said, 'No, not because of those.' I asked, 'Because I was sincere in my adoration?' And God said, 'No.' I then said, 'Because of my pilgrimages and my journeys to acquire knowledge and to enlighten others?' And God again replied, 'No, not because of all this.' So I asked Him, 'O Lord, why then have you forgiven me?' And He answered, 'Do you remember how on a bitterly cold winter day you were walking through the streets of Baghdad and you saw a hungry kitten desperately trying to find shelter from the icy wind, and you had pity on it and picked it up and put it inside your fur and took it into your home?' I said, 'Yes, my Lord, I remember.' And God said, 'Because you were kind to that cat, Abu Bakr, because of that I have forgiven you'" (Schimmel, 1983, p. 16).

Chapter 2

Heresies of the Strategic Approach

The true mystery of the world is the visible, not the invisible.

— Oscar Wilde, *The Picture of Dorian Gray*

We believe that Chapter One has already pointed to the fact that there is a direct conflict between traditional concepts of psychotherapy. It should be clear that one who holds the theoretical perspective presented here is a true "heretic" in terms of classical psychotherapeutic theory and practice. The strategic approach to the treatment of psychic disturbances and behaviors is indeed "heretical" with respect to the majority of psychotherapeutic models. Consequently, before beginning a detailed exposition, we feel that it is important to clearly chart the major points of difference between the strategic approach and the orthodox theories of psychotherapy.

First Heresy: Choose Probability over "Truth"

To know the truth one must imagine myriads of falsehoods. For what is truth? In matters of religion, it is simply the opinion that has survived. In matters of science, it is the ultimate sensation. In matters of art, it is one's last mood.

— Oscar Wilde, *The Artist as Critic*

The therapist who adopts the strategic approach to human problems can appropriately be considered a psychotherapeutic "her-

17

etic" (in the etymological sense of the term, as "one who has
the capacity of choice"), insofar as he or she does not become
entrapped either in a rigid interpretive model of "human nature" or in a stiffly orthodox psychological and psychiatric para-
digm. The strategic approach to therapy, linked directly to
the contemporary philosophy of constructivist knowledge (Bannister and Fransella, 1977; Elster, 1979; Glasersfeld, 1979, 1984;
Foerster, 1970, 1974, 1981, 1984; Kelly, 1955; Maturana, 1978;
Piaget, 1970, 1971; Riedl, 1980; Stolzenberg, 1978; Varela,
1975, 1979; Watzlawick, 1976, 1984) is based on the assertion
of the impossibility—on the part of *any* science—of offering an
absolutely true and definitive explanation of reality. There is
not only one reality but many realities, determined by the perspective of the observer and by the instruments used for observation. From this epistemological perspective, every interpretive
model that presupposes an absolutely true and final explanation of nature and of human behavior is refuted because every
model of this type falls inevitably into the trap of self-referen-
tiality (a sort of naming itself, or self-justification). In the words
of the epistemologist Popper, no theory can find its confirmation within itself or through the means of its own instruments
without avoiding its "nonfalsifiability."* Popper also expresses
succinctly—with the definition of self-sealing theories or propositions—the phenomenon relative to those theoretical models
that protect themselves from falsification: closed all-encompass-
ing systems, in which one finds the explanation for everything.
But precisely because of this characteristic, such theories take
on the role of "religious" conceptions and are thus not models

---

*Since 1931, when Gödel published his famous undecidability theorem using *Prin-
cipia Mathematica* as his basis, we have safely been able to abandon the hope that
any system complex enough to include arithmetic (or, as Tarski has shown, any
language of that complexity) will ever be able to prove its consistency within its
own framework. This proof can only come from the outside, based on additional
axioms, premises, concepts, comparisons, and the like, which the original system itself cannot generate or prove, and which are themselves again only prova-
ble by recourse to a yet wider framework, and so on in an infinite regress of
metasystems, metametasystems, and so forth. In keeping with the basic postu-
lates of *Principia Mathematica,* any statement about a collection (and the proof of
the consistency is one such statement) involves all of the collection and cannot,
must not, therefore, be part of it (Watzlawick, Weakland, and Fisch, 1974, p. 24).

of scientific knowledge. For Bateson (1979), science is a mode of perception, of organizing and giving significance to observations, thereby constructing subjective theories whose value is not definitive.

For the clinician, theories must not be irrefutable truths, but hypotheses related to the world, partial points of view, useful for describing and organizing observable data so as to achieve successful therapies, or to correct unsuccessful ones. Accordingly, it is useful to recall that "it is precisely from the psychologists dedicated to the study of how we know that the notion comes that human beings, insofar as they are 'thinking organisms,' do not operate directly on the reality that they encounter but on the perceptive transformations which form their experience of the world. Therefore, 'categorizations,' 'schemes,' 'attributions,' 'inferences,' 'heuristics,' and conceptualizations constitute the representational systems through which we can realize diverse configurations and explanations of the world. In the same way, for example, a telescope and a radiotelescope offer different representations of the same celestial bodies and their properties" (Selvini-Palazzoli, Cirillo, Selvini, and Fiorentino, 1989, p. 7).

The strategic approach is not based on a theory that describes human nature in terms of the concepts of behavioral and mental "health" or "normality" in opposition to those of pathology, as is the case in traditional theories of psychotherapy. Instead, it is concerned with how humans cope with the problems of existence, with the interaction between individuals, and with the perceptions and relations individuals experience within themselves, with others and with the world. It is not concerned with objects and subjects in and by themselves, but with the object/subject "in relation," since we are convinced of the impossibility of extrapolating a subject from its interactive context. Recall a famous metaphor of Glasersfeld: when we encounter a locked door, that which is of interest to us is not the lock in itself—its nature and intrinsic mechanism—but only the means of finding the key that will open it.

The focus of attention for the strategic therapist is the relation, or, better, the interdependent relations, that each person experiences within self, with others, and with the world. The objective is their functioning, not in general and absolute terms of normality, but in terms of the entirely personal realities that vary from person to person, as well as from context to context.

Therefore the first "heresy" is the passing from "closed" to "open" theoretical systems, from the concept of scientific truth to that of probability; from deterministic linear causality to the more elastic circular causality; from orthodoxy to methodological doubt. In other words, one moves from the fideistic attitude of the believer to the skeptical perspective of the researcher, in the conviction that the fundamental criterion of validation and verification of a therapeutic model is not in its theoretical architecture or the profundity of its analyses, but in its heuristic value and its capacity for authentic intervention, measured in terms of its efficacy and effectiveness in the resolution of the problems to which it is applied.

Second Heresy: Focus on How Rather Than Why

Man is both so perfectible and corruptible that he can go mad by means of his reason.

—G. C. Lichtenberg, *The Little Book of Consolation*

The second heresy of strategic therapy is that the therapist should focus not on the analysis of the deeply rooted or on research into the causes of a problem extrapolated from hidden truths, but rather on the nature of the difficulties facing a subject, couple, or family now, and on how they can be changed. What matters is *process* rather than *content,* the knowledge of *how* rather than *why.* In other words, the role of the therapist is to help the patient to resolve the present problem and to acquire, through this experience, the capacity to adequately confront problems in the future.

The first step is to break the spell. Then the patient learns how to avoid being trapped again by other spells or perceptions and dysfunctional actions. The foundation for this lies in studies and theories that relate to the spontaneous appearance or deliberate realization of change (Watzlawick, Beavin, and Jackson, 1967; Watzlawick, Weakland, and Fisch, 1974). So, it is important to give particular attention to one's perception of reality and to the pragmatic aspects of one's relationship with such reality; to how, by means of these processes, problem situations arise; and finally, to how it is possible, through these same processes, to resolve such problem situations.

Our fundamental assumption is that mental and behavioral disturbances are determined by the subject's perception of reality; by the way the subject perceives (or, better, constructs) a reality, then reacting to it with dysfunctional behavior, or so-called psychopathology. The subject usually believes such behavior to be the best way of dealing with a specific situation. That is to say, frequently it is the "attempted solution" that prolongs or aggravates the problem (Watzlawick, Weakland, and Fisch, 1974).

The therapeutic intervention is represented by the shift from the subject's point of view, from its original rigid and dysfunctional perceptive-reactive position, to an elastic perspective, with more perceptive-reactive possibilities. We return here to the Ethical Imperative established by Foerster: "act always so as to increase the number of choices" (1984, p. 60).

This change in perspective produces a change in the perception of reality, which in turn changes reality itself — the entire situation and the patient's reactions to it.

The subject's perceptions become flexible, and thus can be utilized to confront problematic situations without rigidity and persistent error. The subject acquires the capacity to generate a diversity of possible resolution-strategies when faced with a problem and to begin working toward a solution with the application of the one that appears most likely to effect change. The subject is able to continue the process until a solution is achieved. As Nietzsche stated, "everything that is absolute pertains to pathology"; thus a solution that is successful in one specific situation, when applied to another, can become a complication in the second problem. In fact, the rigid perceptive-reactive system of a troubled person often expresses itself in the obstinate effort to utilize a strategy that seems to resolve the problem — or that in the past did resolve a similar difficulty but that actually reinforces it.

In other words, a rigid perceptive-reactive system can lead to the use of one or more "good solutions" being indiscriminately applied to different problems, with the obvious result that the problems are not only not solved but are complicated by the subject's growing lack of confidence that they can ever be modified. It may seem strange and paradoxical, but often a person's efforts to change either maintain the situation unchanged or increase its complexity. In either case, the person behaves like the drunk who was looking under a lamppost for a key that he had lost; a helpful passerby offered to help him find it. After searching unsuccessfully for quite a while under the lamppost, the helpful gentleman turned to the drunk, a bit annoyed, and asked, "But are you sure that you lost it here?" The other fellow replied, "No, but where I lost it, it is too dark."

Clearly, in light of the foregoing, the first therapeutic action that must be undertaken is to soften the subject's rigid perceptive-reactive system by breaking down both the attempted solutions, which sustain the problem, and the tangle of interpersonal reactions related to them. Then the therapist and client can work toward a cognitive redefinition of both the situation and its effect on the subject.

At this point, we come to another "heresy" in regard to the theoretical and practical orthodoxies in psychotherapy.

Third Heresy: The Therapist Is Responsible

To put reality to the test, one must make it walk a tightrope, and one can judge it only insofar as it becomes acrobatic.

— Oscar Wilde, *The Artist as Critic*

It is clear that a theory about the persistence and the change of human problems that is radically different from classical psychological and psychiatric conceptions leads to *procedures* (strategies designed to provoke change) and *processes* (the evolving phases of change) that are also completely different from classical forms of psychotherapy. At the therapeutic levels of both procedure and process, the strategic approach is the result of the application to the clinical field of the theory of logical types, developed by Whitehead and Russell in their *Principia Mathematica* (1910–1913). It also draws on systems theory and cybernetics (Wiener, 1947; Ashby, 1954, 1956; Bateson, Jackson, Haley, and Weakland, 1956; Bateson and Jackson, 1964; Bateson, 1967, 1972; Foerster, 1974). It is based on the conception of circular causality, the recursion between cause and effect, and the principle of the discontinuity of change and growth. (It is beyond the scope of this chapter to analyze and elucidate these several concepts here, but interested readers are referred to Watzlawick, Beavin, and Jackson, 1967, and Bateson, 1979.)

From this perspective, the usual conviction is that problems that mature over a long period of time necessitate an equally lengthy period of treatment; or that great suffering and complicated situations require a similarly complicated and painful resolution. Thus, we are convinced that a pathological system cannot find the solution to a problem within itself, without running into recursiveness, that is, producing only a so-called first-order, rather than a second-order, change. At this point, we need to digress briefly to distinguish clearly between these two types of change.

There are two types of change: one that occurs within a given system which itself remains unchanged, and one whose occurrence changes the system itself. To exemplify this distinction in more behavioral terms, a person having a nightmare can do many things in his dream — run, hide, fight, scream, jump off a cliff — but no change from any one of these behaviors within the world of the dream would ever terminate the nightmare. We shall henceforth refer to this kind of change as first-order change. The one way out of the nightmare involves a change from dreaming to waking. Waking, obviously, is no longer a part of the dream, but a change to an altogether different state. This kind of change will from now on be referred to as second-order change. This explanation is drawn from *Change: Principles of Problem Formation and Problem Solution* by Watzlawick, Weakland, and Fisch (1974). Indeed, this work represents the basis of our strategic approach and should be read for a full appreciation of its theoretical foundation.

There may be no better example of the strategic approach to the solution of problems (and of its fundamental difference from other forms of psychotherapy) than the famous "nine-dot problem." The problem is to link the nine dots in Figure 2.1 by four straight lines without lifting the pencil from the page. The reader who has never encountered this puzzle should draw the pattern of dots on a piece of paper and try to solve the problem before reading on and, most important, before looking at the solution.

Figure 2.1. The Nine-Dot Problem.

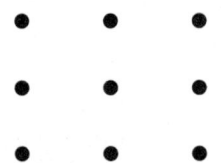

Almost everybody who first tries to solve this problem introduces as part of his problem-solving an assumption which makes the solution impossible. The assumption is that the dots compose a square and that the solution must be found *within* that square — a self-imposed condition which the instructions do not contain. His failure, therefore, does not lie in the impossibility of the task, but in his attempted solution. Having now created the problem, it does not matter in the least which combination of four lines he now tries, and in what order; he always finishes with at least one unconnected dot. This means that he can run through the totality of the first-order change possibilities existing within the square but will not solve the task. The solution is a second-order change which consists in leaving the field and which cannot be contained within itself because, in the language of *Principia Mathematica,* it involves all of a collection and cannot, therefore, be part of it [Watzlawick, Weakland, and Fisch, 1974, p. 39].

To resolve the problem of the nine points, the subject must step outside the logical schema which traps him inside the square.

Very few people manage to solve the nine-dot problem by themselves. Those who fail and give up are usually surprised at the unexpected simplicity of the solution (see Figure 2.2). The analogy between this and many a real-life situation is obvious. We have all found ourselves in comparable boxes, and it did not matter whether we tried to find the solution calmly and logically or, as is more likely, ended up running frantically around in circles. But, as mentioned already, it is only from inside the box, in the first-order change perspective, that the solution appears as a surprising flash of enlightenment beyond our control. In the second-order change perspective it is a simple change from one set of premises to another of the same logical type. The one set includes the rule that the task must be solved within the [assumed] square; the other does not. In other words, the solution is found as a result of examining the assumptions *about* the dots, not the dots themselves. Or, to make the same statement in more philosophical terms, it obviously makes a difference whether we consider ourselves as pawns in a game whose rules we call reality or as players of the game who know that the rules are "real" only to the extent that we have created or accepted them, and we can change them [Watzlawick, Weakland, and Fisch, 1974, p. 25].

Figure 2.2. Solution to the Nine-Dot Problem.

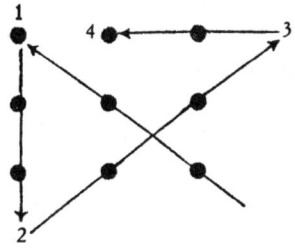

At this point it may be useful to compare this kind of problem-solving and change with the assumptions that are at the root of most classical schools of psychotherapy. It is generally held that change comes about through insight into the past causes which are responsible for present trouble. But, as the nine-dot problem exemplifies, there is no cogent reason for this excursion into the past; the genesis of the self-defeating assumption which precedes the solution is quite irrelevant; the problem is solved in the here and now by stepping outside the "box." There is increasing awareness among clinicians that while insight may provide very sophisticated explanations of a symptom, it does little if anything to change it for the better.

This empirical fact raises an important epistemological issue. All theories have limitations which follow logically from their premises. In the case of psychiatric theories, these limitations are more often than not attributed to human nature. For instance, within the psychoanalytic framework, symptom removal without the solution of the underlying conflict responsible for the symptom must lead to symptom substitution. This is not because this complication lies in the nature of the human mind; it lies in the nature of the theory, that is, in the conclusions that follow from its premises [Watzlawick, Weakland, and Fisch, 1974, p. 26].

From this perspective, human problems can be resolved by means of specific strategies that break the feedback loops that maintain the problem. Change in the subject's behavior and insight follow from this breakdown of a dysfunctional equilibrium, because change depends on modification of the perceptive-reactive system — or the view of reality — which is actively maintained by the "attempted solutions" applied by the subject. The patient must be "forced" to abandon his rigid perspective and be led to other possible perspectives that can bring about new "realities" and new solutions, as in the example of the nine-dot problem.

To achieve such a result, one need not search for a presupposed "original trauma," the removal of which would solve the patient's problems; neither is a slow and progressive acquisition of insight indispensable to the search for self-consciousness. These are procedures based on assumptions of a linear causality — of a deterministic relationship between cause and effect, as well as conceptions and convictions, among others — which have been overcome by modern science, from biology to physics.

Instead of linear assumptions, what is needed are direct and indirect behavior prescriptions, paradoxical interventions, suggestions, and reframing. They break through the rigidity of the relational and cognitive system that maintains the problem situation and they complete the indispensable logical leap that opens up of new ways of change, making possible both personal growth and a new psychological equilibrium. As Milton Erickson affirms (Watzlawick, Weakland, and Fisch, 1974, p. ix):

> Psychotherapy is sought not primarily for enlightenment about the unchangeable past but because of dissatisfaction with the present and a desire to better the future. In what direction and how much change is needed neither the patient nor the therapist can know. But a change in the current situation is required, and once established, however small, necessitates other minor changes, and a snowballing effect of these minor changes leads to other more significant changes in accord with the patient's potentials. Whether the changes are evanescent, permanent, or evolve into other more significant changes is of vital importance in any understanding of human behavior for the self and others. I have viewed much of what I have done as expediting the current of change already seething within the person and family — but currents that need the "unexpected," the "illogical," and the "sudden" move to lead them into tangible fruition.

In this absolutely heretical approach the therapist assumes the responsibility of directly influencing the behavior and worldview of the patient. To this end, in the interests of the patient, he uses communicative strategies and other means of effecting change. This point will be dealt with at length in Chapter Four, but for the moment all that is necessary is to clarify these points:

1. In strategic therapy, the therapist maintains the initiative in all that takes place during the course of treatment and applies a specific technique to deal with each particular problem. For the therapist, the first question must always be, Which strategy functions best in a given case?

2. If a specific therapy is functioning correctly, certain indicators of change should appear early on in the treatment. If this is not the case, most likely the intervention chosen is not appropriate and must be superseded with another that is more successful.

3. The therapist must possess a mental elasticity and a wide repertory of strategies and techniques which, as we shall see, stem from different orientations than those of the classical schools of psychotherapy. There must be room to shift gears when the facts make it clear that one is far from the desired goal, and to study ad hoc strategies so that techniques already successfully utilized in similar cases can be creatively modified. As we have been stressing, the therapist needs to adapt the treatment to the patient, not the patient to the treatment.

Fourth Heresy: Change Comes *Before* Insight

It is much more difficult to do a thing than to talk about it.

—Oscar Wilde, *The Artist as Critic*

Another heresy at the level of strategies and processes of change lies in the fact that most psychotherapies, imbued with the idea of *cogito-centrism* (the centrality of thought in respect to action), have as their point of departure the presupposition that action follows from thought. Consequently, to change distorted behavior or a problematical situation, the patient's thinking must change first. Hence the necessity of insight, of procedures to analyze the mind, and all those techniques based on "consciousness raising" and "rationalization" of action.

In strategic therapy — based on radical constructivism — this process is inverted. We believe that in order to change a problem situation one must first change the action and *then* change the patient's thinking — or, better, the point of view or "frame of reality." Foerster and his Aesthetic Imperative again come to mind in this regard.

It is our concrete experience that determines any change in our manner of perceiving and reacting to reality. We believe that the entire work of Jean Piaget clearly demonstrates how the acquisition of new knowledge occurs through a process that moves *from experience to cognition.* Only after change — or the new experience — is achieved does cognition allow it to be repeated and reapplied at will.

We do not, therefore, want to negate the influence of thought and cognition on action, but we do wish to emphasize that change of a perceptive-reactive situation must originate first in concrete experience; only after that can it become cognitive knowledge. By *experience* we do not mean the reductive physical concept of sensory-motor action, but rather that which we all perceive in our relations with others and with the world. A strong emotion determined by a relation or communication with another person may be an example of a new, concrete situation and can shift the patient's outlook on reality. A casual disruption in our usual routine or a strong suggestion are other examples of concrete experiences that can change our frame of reality.

The strategic therapist is, therefore, oriented pragmatically to action and to the rupture of dysfunctional feedbacks that the patient experiences within, with others, and with the world. The aim is to effect this change by bringing about concrete perceptive-reactive experiences. The therapist first seeks to produce modifications of the subject's perceptive-active faculty and then to pass on to redefinitions, at the cognitive level, of that which is experienced, in a pragmatic synthesis of the therapist's influence and the patient's continuous wish for autonomy. From this perspective, any attempt to produce insight at the early stage of therapy is considered to be a counterproductive maneuver insofar as it increases resistance to change. Every system, according to the principle of homeostasis, resists any alteration of itself. As we shall see, the rupture of the perceptive-reactive system and attempted solutions must usually occur without the patient's awareness of the process—this to obviate resistance. Only after successfully effecting the change can the therapist explain the "tricks" or the "benevolent lies" utilized.

To make clearer the differences between the ways *procedure* and *process* are used in strategic therapy and in other approaches, let us use a clinical example: Confronted with an agoraphobic patient, traditional psychotherapy would begin by exploring the origin of the patient's fear and its causes in the past. Then the patient would be led, by means of rationalization and explanation, to confront the fear and its triggers. Normally, this procedure requires many months or even years.

In strategic therapy, a patient may be asked to perform some embarrassing task when experiencing attacks of anxiety or panic, with the usual result that the person comes to the next appointment feeling guilty for not having carried out the assignment but—oddly—also noting that in the interim the symptoms that brought the person to therapy have not recurred. By means of a "benevolent lie" that leads the person to behave differently, the rigid system of perception that had restricted the patient to a symptomatic response is shattered. From that point on, the person—whether aware of it or not—has experienced mastery of what had seemed an overwhelming fear, and the treatment begins to make progress. Through a concrete personal experience, the patient has acquired faith in the possibility of modifying the situation.

To return to the initial concept, it is action or experience that produces change, which is then strengthened and made conscious.

Strategic therapy, then, can be seen as a chess game played between therapist and patient. After each "change" or result, one proceeds to a redefinition of change itself. The therapeutic program develops strategy after strategy, based on the effects observed in the effort, to apply the most efficacious treatment for a specific problem or a specific phase of therapy.

In a chess game particular combinations of moves and countermoves follow from a specific opening made by one player. In therapy, there are particular strategic programs for specific types of problems (in Chapter Five we shall give two examples). Often the therapist must creatively modify the system of foreseeable moves by finding new, unexpected, and apparently illogical strategies that take into account the whole gamut of possible combinations, thus amplifying the complexity of the game and its possibilities. Thus the strategic approach is not a simple series of effective "recipes," but a prospect for confronting human problems. It is not concerned with extinguishing all problems in the life of the patient, but with finding solutions to the specific problem that the patient is coping with at this time. The idea is not to apply magical tricks, but rather to creatively adapt, to each particular individual and context, logical principles concerning the formation and solution of problems.

The process of therapy closes with the "checkmate" of the problem presented at its outset, and with the patient's acquisition of the "procedures" to autonomously play and win this specific sort of game. For the rest, says Bateson, to live is to play "a game whose purpose is to discover the rules, which are always changing and always undiscoverable" (1972, pp. 19–20).

Chapter 3

The Development
of the Strategic Approach

*In order to observe the most simple, but real, relations
amongst things, it is necessary to have a deep knowledge.
And it is not strange that only extraordinary men make
those discoveries, that then appear so easy and simple.*

—G. C. Lichtenberg, *The Little Book of Consolation*

In order to define the quintessentials of the strategic approach
to psychotherapy we need to explore both its origins and its
modern-day applications. First, rather than simply explore the
origins of this specific curative art, we should perhaps examine
the whole tradition of "strategic thought," whose roots extend
deep into the history of mankind. By *strategic thought* we do not
mean a specific philosophical school of thought but rather a
thought approach, or, more specifically, "liberal thinking," which
by virtue of its fundamental elasticity negates the existence of
any form of "absolute" or unquestionable "truth." In this way
this approach allows for a pragmatic and clear-minded analysis of how things in the world work. Referred to as "radical constructivism," it dates back to the Hellenic tradition of Epicurus
through to those of the pre-Socratic philosophers and the Sophists
and, in the Oriental world, it forms the basis for certain behavioral dictates of Buddhism and Zen.

By means of the voices and personalities of many of the
world's great thinkers, this approach to thought has colored the
cultural heritage of the entire human race, from the primeval
era right up to the present day, and, needless to say, this historical and philosophical perspective itself merits far greater attention than either the competence of the authors or the limits of
this text allow.

Moving away from the historical perspective, we will now look at recent applications of "strategic" or "constructivist" thought to behavioral and mental disorders. From this perspective, Milton Erickson can undoubtedly be considered to be the father of strategic therapy. Throughout his brilliant, forty-year-long career as hypnotherapist and psychotherapist, Erickson employed countless strategies and techniques in the speedy resolution of both the behavioral and mental disorders of his patients.

Erickson, after having become the leading authority in both the study and practice of hypnosis, then ingeniously transferred his discoveries and observations relative to hypnosis and suggestion to the clinical field. This met with great success, particularly with regard to the effectiveness of certain patterns of language and other forms of therapeutic communication capable of inducing rapid and effective changes within the patient.

In fact, the element that until recently has been neglected in Erickson's work is the strategic approach he outlined for the treatment of single patients, couples, and families, without prior trance induction. While not involving hypnosis per se, the therapy clearly reveals Erickson's underlying conception of hypnosis as a relational and psychosocial phenomenon. For the first time it was free of its traditional aura of mystery and "magic ritual," but was effected through a particular style of therapeutic communication based on refined forms of verbal and nonverbal language. Erickson never formulated a theory of "human nature" or of "personality," as for him every person was a unique being, with completely individual ways of perceiving and elaborating reality and therefore with a personal history. Even the clinical study of an individual should take this into account, he believed, with therapeutic strategies always adapted to the patient's individual personality, relational context, and life experiences.

As Haley observes (1973), strategic therapy is not a particular conception or theory; it is a name for those types of therapeutic interventions in which the psychotherapist assumes the responsibility of influencing people directly. The Ericksonian perspective has no restricting theoretical prejudices, nor any rigid conceptualizations that claim to exhaustively describe human nature, but this approach is nonetheless closely connected with system-oriented communication theory and family therapy. Although Erickson, essentially a pragmatist rather than a theorist, did not leave any formal description of his personal model of psychotherapy, it can be deduced from the content of the numerous articles and studies on hypnosis that he published during his career. His particular techniques and strategies, or, if you prefer, his personal attitude to therapy, is itself the best concrete illustration of his strategic approach. Many authors have interpreted it according to their own personal theoretical and practical frameworks (Bandler and Grinder, 1975a; Bergman, 1985; Haley, 1967, 1973, 1985; Lankton and Lankton, 1983; Rabkin, 1977; Ritterman, 1983; Rosen, 1982; Erickson, Rossi, and Rossi, 1979; Erickson and Rossi, 1982; Simon, Stierlin, and Wynne, 1985; Watzlawick, 1978, 1985; Zeig, 1980, 1985, 1987). As far as they are concerned, it is therefore probably more appropriate to talk of "Ericksonian-inspired" therapy than of Ericksonian therapy in the strict sense.

Erickson's work embraces the development and systematization of communication from an interactional or pragmatic perspective, and it is this to which we refer when we use the term *strategic therapy*. In fact, the strategic model derives from an evolutionary synthesis of all the various branches of systems theory, the study of the family and of communication carried out by what has become known as the Palo Alto Group under Bateson and Jackson, and Erickson's work.

As the cybernetician Foerster maintains (1981), the "Copernican" revolution of the 1950s in the fields of psychology and psychiatry, aptly described as "systemic-interactional," was not brought about solely by the work of clinical psychologists. It was also the fruit of the cross-fertilization of exciting discoveries in various scientific disciplines: in anthropology, with Bateson's communication studies; in cybernetics and physics, with the theory of Ashby, Foerster, and others; and in the studies of clinical hypnosis by Erickson.

As Haley affirms (1973), apart from being the father of strategic therapy, Erickson also provided the technical inspiration for the development of many of the therapeutic procedures employed in systemic family therapy. And, while Bateson is the father of the systemic-interactional perspective in both psychology and psychiatry, it is Erickson who excels in practical clinical procedures and the speedy solution of psychological problems. His professional life was dedicated to research and the clinical application of his intuitive insights and ideas. These led to a treasury of intervention techniques, which continue to be the basic therapeutic tools of most strategic therapists today. So, to return to the theoretical development of strategic therapy, the psychological model that has been presented here could also logically be called "systemic-strategic," inasmuch as we hold the Palo Alto Group's approach to systemic therapy to be completely compatible with, and complementary to, Erickson's operational procedures. So revolutionary were the new discoveries and experiences of the fifties, sixties, and seventies that they led to the development of a whole new concept of reality and of a person's perception of reality — and, as a natural consequence of this, to a new way of looking at problem formation and problem resolution. Unfortunately, space limitations do not allow us to explore more than just a few aspects of this practical-theoretical development.

The Systemic Revolution in Therapy

Looking at the development of systems theory and its successive application in psychotherapy, it becomes evident that, in common with other scientific conceptualizations, the classical psychological and psychiatric theories are steeped in the epistemology of their time and possess "all the unmistakable characteristics of a theory based on the first law of thermodynamics, with its almost exclusive emphasis on the phenomena of conservation and transformation of energy. . . . The concept of causality underlying this model is of necessity a linear, unidirectional one, whereby event *A* effects (determines) event *B*, whose occurrence, in turn, is the cause of event *C*, and so on, from the past through the present and into the future" (Watzlawick and Weakland, 1977, p. XII). It therefore follows that, by approaching the investigation or explanation of an event from this perspective, one is compelled to analyze past events in order to understand and explain present ones and so be able to induce the changes necessary to solve a patient's problems. But around 1950, a different epistemology began to gain ground in scientific circles. This, "rather than being based on the concept of energy and on the subsequent unidirectional causality, is based on the concept of information — that is to say order, model, negative entropy — namely, on the second law of thermodynamics. Its principles are cybernetic, its causality is of a circular type, of retroactive nature, and the period of time, in which information makes it the main element, is directed to communication processes of systems intended in a wider sense, and, therefore, human systems as well, for example, families, vast organizations, and even international relations" (Watzlawick, 1976, p. 8).

   If you observe the behavior of individuals from the systemic and cybernetic point of view, that is to say, if you consider personal entities as not standing on their own and having their own "determined" evolutive and behavioral scheme, but see them interacting inside a system of relationships or a context characterized by a continuous and mutual exchange of information between single entities that influence one another, the classical view of personality and human behavior studies is completely modified. To analyze a person in monadic isolation, and not in relation to other people and within a specific context, leads nowhere. Just as in mathematics a number exists only in relation to its function in an operational context and in its relation with other numbers, the single person's self-expression is in relation to interactions with other people and the surrounding environment. We must add to this general consideration the concept of *retroaction,* the peculiarity of all human beings inside a communication system not to be mere transmitters or information targets, but to always give and receive a retroaction (feedback) in response to the message transmitted or received. The retroaction is the return message to the transmitter that establishes a chain of information and mutual influences between transmitter and receiver. By means of the retroaction, a kind of circular causality is formed, inside of which are not only a relationship of cause and effect between the first transmitter of the message and the receiver, but a more complex form of mutual cause involving all the elements of their relationship. In this way people overcome the deterministic concepts of unidirectionality and linear causality, which can be graphically shown as follows:

A————————▶B————————▶C————————▶D

In opposition to this linear, deterministic view of causality stands the modern perspective, based on the concept of a circular (feedback) causality, as exemplified by the following figure:

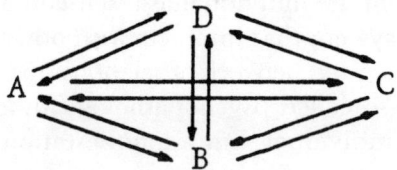

Here every component of the system is linked to all the others by reverberating circuits. Once such a circular process has been established, one can no longer talk about origins and results, causes and effects. The system must be studied in its totality, for the whole is more than, and different from, the mere sum total of its parts. Any attempt to study the components in isolation would destroy the totality and would produce results that are of no help for our understanding of the system. Rather, the opposite is now the case: our understanding of any *one* component or function of the system presupposes our understanding of the system as a whole.

This perspective has important implications for the understanding of psychological and psychiatric phenomena, which until recently were conceived as purely intrapsychic factors and the result of unidirectional and strictly deterministic processes running from the past into the present. In adopting this different view, our approach reoriented itself toward the innovative, system-oriented perspective already adopted in most branches of the social and behavioral sciences.

Gregory Bateson was undoubtedly the inspiration behind this shift in conceptualization, and, together with Don D. Jackson, formulated and practiced therapy in this way. The Bateson-

Jackson team transferred the principles of cybernetics and anthropology to the study of families with an emotionally disturbed member. Thus was systemic family therapy born: a combination of empirical results with a simultaneous shift in theoretical perspective — from the classical psychiatric viewpoint, which analyzes abnormal behavior within a clinical diagnostic framework, to an anthropological perspective, which seeks to explain the function and workings of that aberrant behavior within its own specific context. A hypothesis evolved into theory, namely, that the key to mental disorder lies in dysfunctional communications between patients and others surrounding them. Attention was shifted away from the individual as a self-contained unit to the individual as a system that interacts with other systems within a complexly structured network of relationships. In this perspective, therefore, so-called psychopathological behavior is not a problem of the individual, but a manifestation of pathological interaction between individuals.

Thus psychotherapy shifted from the "intrapsychic" to the "relational" approach. It changed from being retrospective to studying events in the here and now, from the "why" of a problem toward its "what" and its potential solution. The therapist was no longer a passive element in the therapeutic relationship, but an active agent bringing personal influence to bear through practical interventions. Thus therapy came to be defined as the careful study of patterns of interpersonal communication, followed by changes in the dysfunctional relationship patterns in the patient's family by means of direct interventions or prescriptions of a paradoxical and often seemingly illogical nature.

Careful studies of communication patterns enable the researcher to identify those that may lead to pathogenic forms of interaction. If, for instance, a person is given a message that contains two contradictory — mutually exclusive — orders, and if that person cannot leave the interactional context, the result will be some form of disturbed behavior. This is a typical example of the famous "double bind" concept, which Bateson had found to be present in the communication of disturbed families. Individuals trapped in such a communication pattern are bound to experience contradictions and guilt, no matter how they react to the messages they receive, since these messages are structured in such a way that they leave no way out that will not provoke anxiety and guilt. These double binds have been seen to have, as Giannattasio and Nencini (1983) observed, considerable heuristic power, that is, a strong prognostic quality and not merely a confirmatory, retrospective value, like so many other concepts in psychotherapy.

The research group headed by Bateson and Jackson (the latter being both the founder and first director of the Mental Research Institute [MRI] of Palo Alto, California) also showed how other patterns of interaction can produce effects similar to that of the double bind: tactics, games, symmetry, complementarity, and other communications can induce a person, usually the most fragile of the group, to develop "psychopathological" behavior. A particular model of family treatment evolved from these empirical observations and their interpretation, based entirely on therapeutic interventions designed to block such self-reinforcing patterns within a malfunctioning communication system. These techniques often incorporate the use of paradoxical messages, as do "symptom prescriptions" and other procedures, such as therapeutic double binds.

In addition, two of the more revolutionary innovations taken from systems theory into clinical practice are the use of the one-way mirror and the videorecording of therapy sessions. Both continue to enjoy considerable success, which only goes to stress the methodological and epistemological strength of the systemic approach as a tool for both research and therapy. The recording of sessions and the use of the one-way mirror enable members of the team who are not in the treatment room to observe the session, and to intervene by offering advice to the therapist over the telephone. Thus, in effect, therapy is not carried out by one therapist alone, but by a consultative group as a whole. When therapy is observed by a team of therapists it is rendered more effective. Moreover, a videorecording provides not only a permanent record of the session but also the best possible basis for retrospective analysis.

It will be clear at this point just how different from other models of psychotherapy this procedure is, both in its therapeutic application and in the context of clinical research. Indeed, in all the other forms of therapy it is absolutely out of the question to intrude upon the session, and the only record of what took place is the therapist's personal account. Despite the best will in the world, therapists are likely to highlight details that are of greatest interest to their own research and most in line with the theories that form their points of reference. Inevitably they will discount a great portion of the session as being of little value. Anyone involved in scientific observation knows how difficult it is to collect data in an objective way, even when observing a situation from the outside; it goes without saying how much more difficult this is for an observer who is personally involved in the therapeutic encounter. Thus, "participative observation" is often subject to considerable distortion as regards the relevance of the data, and instead is frequently used to support the therapist's own theories. To paraphrase Einstein, it is the theory that determines what we can observe.

The success of the systemic model lies in its utilization of empirical observations of both the family and the therapeutic interaction. Thus rigorous epistemological criteria form the basis of systemic therapy, along with research procedures utilizing recent advances in the philosophy of science and methods that set it apart from most other psychological and psychiatric models.

From Family Therapy to Strategic Therapy

After this brief look at the birth and evolution of systemic therapy the reader will appreciate how much these theories and methods relate to Erickson's studies of hypnosis and his mode of clinical practice. And, as we have said earlier, particularly with regard to the strategies of change, there is unquestionably a link between the great hypnotist's work and that of the Palo Alto group (MRI).

It should be pointed out that Bateson, Haley, and Weakland, while engaged in their famous project on communication, studied not only Erickson's techniques in great depth but also his ideas regarding mental problems in general. At that time

Erickson was at the peak of his career as a hypnotherapist. His fame stemmed above all from his almost miraculous therapeutic successes achieved with the use of most uncommon strategies, which were decidedly at odds with classical psychotherapeutic procedures. They were so original and effective and efficient that Erickson quickly gained a reputation as a "quasi magician." Predictably, criticism and disapproval rained down on Erickson from all sectors of traditional medicine and psychiatry throughout the United States.

The founders of systemic therapy based themselves on Erickson's methods, and as their approach evolved, it became clear that Erickson had, in fact, both formulated and applied many of the therapeutic strategies that Bateson and Jackson later formalized as integral parts of their systemic model. For example, on the basis of his experience with hypnosis, Erickson had already used paradoxical prescriptions (therapeutic double binds); he utilized surprise and the "use of resistance" as therapeutic techniques; and, just as a great magician might do, he would put the patient in such a position that taking the only possible way out of the dilemma solved the problem. Therefore, through his use of hypnosis, Erickson arrived at a form of therapy that was congruent with systemic therapy as it was developing at the time in the United States and overseas, a therapy which yielded exceptional results for single individuals, couples, and families, and all in a shorter time than was usual until then.

Strategic therapy focuses attention on the definition of the patient's problem, the identification of the behavior that maintains the problem, and, most important, on seeking ways to modify the situation in the shortest time possible. In this, it differs from classical systemic family therapy, which concentrates on family interaction and its reorganization. But it must also be said that often the two approaches overlap and complement each other. In fact, solving the problem that the patient presents usually brings about changes in family interaction, just as modifications in the family system can lead to the solution of the patient's problem. The fundamental question for the therapist is which of the many strategies available would be the most effective. From this decision will flow specifics, such as whether to meet the patient alone or with other family members, and whether to intervene directly in the family system or, after reaching an understanding of the family's interaction, to concentrate on the identified patient.

It should be pointed out that there is no one definitive model of strategic therapy; in fact, numerous different models of therapy have evolved under the banner of "the strategic approach." However, there are two models that, more than any others, have influenced the theory and practice of strategic therapists: one is identified with Haley (1967, 1973, 1976), Montalvo and Haley (1973), and Madanes (1981); the other is the MRI model (Weakland, Fisch, Watzlawick, and Bodin, 1974; Watzlawick, Weakland, and Fisch, 1974; Watzlawick, 1978; Herr and Weakland, 1979; Fisch, Weakland, and Segal, 1982). Both models have emerged out of the experiences of those who both were part of Bateson's original group and worked closely with Milton Erickson. These experiences formed the bases of their own work and research as therapists and led them to formalize the two strategic approaches. Strategic and systemic therapy are, in many ways, in tune with one another, but they differ in a few theoretical and practical particulars.

For Haley and his colleagues the main problems are the hierarchical incongruities within the family and their pathological effects involving coalitions and power plays. They see the symptom as a metaphor for the problem and also as its pseudosolution by the patient. The therapy concentrates on the management of power within the family (the symptoms themselves are regarded as instruments of power) and on reorganizing the hierarchy. By so doing, it changes the whole power structure. The therapist joins in the family's power game in order to restructure it along more functional lines (Haley, 1976, p. 80).

As Madanes observes (1981), one way to understand the approach is to think of it as giving instructions that point directly at the target; for example, the therapist might tell a parent to take a reluctant child to school. Sometimes the therapist's direct intervention will not have any effect. In that case, the therapist offers an alternative strategy to try to stimulate the family to achieve the objective. If the second effort does not produce the desired effect, the therapist tries again, with another idea.

This approach is markedly directive and is based on the idea that it is essential to overcome the crises that arise at the various stages in a family's development, which Haley (1973) has identified as a sequence of six:

1. Courtship
2. Early marriage
3. Birth of a child and parent/child relationship
4. Midmarriage
5. Child's leaving the parental home
6. Retirement and old age

Of particular interest to the strategic approach is the period when the grown-up child leaves home. It is generally assumed that the serious pathological phenomena (schizophrenia, delinquency, drug addiction, and the like) that often manifest themselves at this stage in a young person's life are often due to the difficulties attendant on realizing that a particular chapter of life has come to an end. In fact, all the traditional diagnostic categories, considered in the context of the family situation of the individual, are redefined in terms of difficulties in developing from one stage to another in the life cycle (Madanes, 1981).

Within the framework of strategic therapy, problems or symptoms are seen as modes of interpersonal communication in a specific social context, while the pathological systems are described by Haley in terms of malfunctioning hierarchies that need to be reorganized. MRI, however, maintains that a problem is caused by the action-reaction mechanism that is set in motion and maintained by the attempted solutions the patient adopts to cope with his problems. Consequently, therapy should focus on the cycle of interactions that maintain or even worsen the problem. The therapist has to interrupt these repetitive patterns of malfunctioning interaction and replace them with less dysfunctional ones. Clearly, the patient's conceptualization of the problem and attempts at solving it are essential, because the therapist relies heavily on them as well as on details of others' reactions to these attempted solutions. These diagnostic data dictate the therapist's choice of interventions.

The MRI group maintains that even the smallest change effected within a rigid system causes a chain reaction that eventually modifies the whole system. As Hoffman (1981) said, MRI's Brief Therapy Project is characterized by its elegant parsimony: "If a clinician is successful in identifying the sequence of which the symptom is a vital part, a very small change can presumably be pinpointed accurately enough to have a wide-reaching effect" (p. 213). Since this approach and the strategies it employs are oriented toward minimal goals, they noticeably reduce the patient's resistance to change.

The therapist's actions are subtle and disguised, seemingly nondirective and modest. Most of the prescriptions are oriented toward apparently banal goals, but in reality are designed to bring about real, tangible change in the patient's behavior.

To conclude, we have seen that in the Haley and MRI approaches, very often the same therapeutic procedures, typical of the strategic approach, are directed at different foci depending on different authors' conceptions as to what precisely perpetuates the problem. The therapeutic model presented here is based on the fruits of more than twenty years of implementation of systems- and communication-based therapies; it owes a great deal to recent research into the effectiveness and efficiency of strategies aimed at changing problem situations.

Chapter 4

Clinical Practice, Processes, and Procedures

*I certainly can't say that change is always for the better;
but what I can say is that improvement necessitates
change.*

—G. C. Lichtenberg, *The Little Book of Consolation*

Before we move on to examine the clinical application of our
approach to therapy, it will be useful to review a few of its basic
concepts. The relationship between therapists and patients in
strategic therapy is not a sort of "paid friendship" and is far from
being a form of "consolation" or "confession." Rather, as we have
seen, it is a kind of chess game between therapists on the one
hand and patients with their problems on the other. As in chess,
there is a set of rules, step-by-step development, and a series
of consolidated strategies, each appropriate to a specific situation—all designed to bring a game to a satisfactory conclusion.

In this chapter, we will explain the therapeutic "process"
step by step (much as a chess manual explains possible moves),
from the first encounter between therapist and patient, right
through to the end of treatment. The chapter will be punctu-
ated with a series of detailed descriptions of both consolidated
strategies and therapeutic techniques—analogous to the common opening moves in a chess game. Clearly, we cannot be exhaustive as regards the repertoire of possible strategies, any more
than a chess manual can detail all possible moves. The combinations in both cases are infinite, depending on the interaction
between the two players.

It is important to point out that the analogy between chess
and therapy falls down in one important particular: that of the

45

fundamentally different natures of the two types of "game." Chess is a "zero-sum" game (Neumann and Morgenstern, 1944), a game that necessarily has a winner and a loser, while therapy is a "non-zero-sum" game, in which either both players win or both lose. In fact, if the therapist succeeds in overcoming the patient's resistance to change and solves the presenting problem, both players emerge winners — the therapist, whose professionalism is intact, and the patient, whose problems are solved or under control. Should the therapy fail, however, both are losers: the patient's problems remain unsolved and the therapist is frustrated by what seems to be professional inadequacy. For this reason, we maintain that whatever the strategy the therapist adopts in order to win the game as quickly as possible, even if those means seem manipulative or cynical, the strategy is legitimate from an ethical standpoint.

Processes and Procedures of Therapy

Strategic therapy is usually accomplished in twenty sessions or less, and is directed at the elimination of symptoms and the resolution of problems. This approach, as will become clear, is not behaviorist in nature, nor is it a superficial, symptom-oriented therapy. As we have said, the success of strategic therapy in resolving a problem lies in breaking the circular reaction system that maintains the problem, redefining the situation, and subsequently changing the patient's perception of the reality that is forcing the adoption of dysfunctional solutions. In this sense, the past and clinical history of the patient serve only to inform the selection of strategies with which to tackle the problem; they do not form the basis per se of the therapeutic procedure, as in the case of psychoanalysis. From the first meeting with the patient, instead of concentrating on the past, the therapist focuses on, and evaluates, the following:

1. What is happening within the three types of the patient's interdependent relationships, namely, with self, with others, and with the world
2. How the problem presented is perpetuated within those relationship patterns

3. How the patient has tried so far to solve the problem (what the attempted solution is)
4. How the problem situation can be changed as quickly as possible

After having formulated one or more hypotheses relating to these four points, and having reached an agreement with the patient(s) regarding the goal of therapy, the therapist can put the various strategies into operation.

If the treatment is effective, there is usually a lessening of the symptoms right from the first session, followed by a progressive change in the patient's way of perceiving self, others, and the world around. The patient's rigid perceptual framework, which maintained the problem, gradually becomes more elastic. At the same time, the patient's sense of autonomy and self-esteem increase, along with the realization that solving the problems is now a tangible possibility. The following list of the stages of treatment helps to delineate the processes involved in this form of strategic therapy (adapted from Weakland, Fisch, Watzlawick, and Bodin, 1974, and Nardone, 1988):

1. First appointment and building of therapeutic relationship
2. Definition of the problem
3. Agreement on the goals of treatment
4. Pinpointing the perceptive-reactive system keeping the problem alive
5. Devising therapy and change strategies
6. Conclusion of treatment

Each of these stages will be explored in detail, and specific examples can be found in the case histories in the concluding chapters.

First Appointment and Building of the Therapeutic Relationship

The initial meeting between therapist and patient is of great importance to the therapy as a whole; even Aristotle said that a good start was half the job already done. In this opening phase of therapy, the primary goal is to create a positive atmosphere of trust within which the therapist can collect information that will be of use in formulating a diagnosis and preparing the ground for subsequent interventions. Here it is fundamental to learn to speak the patient's language; in other words, the therapist must fit into the representational framework of the person seeking help, adapting personal language and actions to the "world image" and communicative style of the patient. For example, if the patient is a rational, logical person, the therapist should speak and act in logical and rational ways, with no flights of fancy. If, however, the therapist is confronted with an imaginative and poetic person, then imaginative and creative language — not rigid, logical rationality — will put the therapist in tune with the patient. Clearly, this initial step is completely contrary to the usual psychoanalytic procedures, in which it is the patient who has to learn the language of psychoanalysis and become conversant with its theories in order to benefit from therapy.

This first stage is critical. By accepting what patients communicate about themselves and their problems and by speaking each patient's language, the therapist can create that atmosphere of trust, understanding, and positive influence that will allow "manipulation" and guidance of the patient's actions. In effect, the therapist assumes therapeutic power and overcomes the patient's resistance to change.

A good therapist, in this first contact with the patient, stimulates the patient's motivation and trust, giving positive suggestions and leading the patient, without contradicting the patient's convictions, to carry out actions that may be completely at odds with the patient's prior conceptual framework.

Defining the Problem

Successfully resolving the problem and the dysfunctional interactional system by which it is maintained requires that it be clearly and concretely defined. Right from the first session, the therapist must concentrate on the problem itself. Arriving at a pragmatic definition requires not only taking into consideration the patient's personal observations but also eliciting from the patient the clearest possible explanation of the problem. This process can take some time, as people often are not good at describing their problems clearly, and it may become necessary to look more closely at what the patient is experiencing in order to help define the problem and move on to the practical part of the treatment. That this process can be time-consuming should not worry the therapist unduly, because the sessions spent in clarifying the problem, if conducted in the patient's own communicative style, constitute a form of therapeutic intervention. Even as early as this exploratory stage, it is not unusual to see symptoms improve. The famous "Hawthorne Effect," well known to social psychologists, describes this phenomenon exactly (Mayo, 1933): simply knowing that someone is concerned can positively influence the situation. Moreover, a clear and concrete definition of the problem is of great help in finding the fastest and most effective solution, and thus time spent in the so-called diagnostic phase will be made up for later.

In defining and evaluating the problem, the therapist should bear in mind a few general characteristics of human problems that will help in the definition of specific situations. Greenberg (1980) formulated two categories of human problems: (a) a person's relationship with himself, and (b) a person's relationship with others. We would like to add a third category: (c) a person's relationship with the world — that is, with the social environment, the values and norms of the social context within which the person lives.

In our view, if difficulties arise in one of these relationship areas, the others are also affected. In fact, all three types of relationship, components of the existence of every individual, influence each other and interact to the extent that they are interdependent.

What seems to be most important in this problem-based therapy is to establish how this circularity of interdependence works and whether problems in one of the three relationship dimensions are more keenly felt by the patient than those in others. In such a case, the dimension in question would provide the ideal starting point for interventions through which the whole dysfunctional perceptive-reactive system could eventually be changed.

In order to arrive at a concrete definition of the problem the therapist needs to be able to answer the following questions:

- What are the patient's usual, observable behavior patterns?
- How does the patient define the problem?
- How does the problem manifest itself?
- In whose company does the problem appear, worsen, disguise itself, or not appear?
- Where does it usually appear?
- In what situations?
- How often does the problem appear and how serious is it?
- What has been done and is currently being done (by the patient alone or by others) to resolve the problem?
- Whom or what does the problem benefit?
- Who could be hurt by the disappearance of the problem?

We believe that, having answered these questions, the therapist is able to select and put into effect the appropriate strategies aimed at breaking the vicious circle of action and reaction that maintains the problem.

Agreement on the Goals of Therapy

The necessity of defining the goals of therapy may appear obvious, but we consider it of great pragmatic importance for two main reasons: (1) it is a guide for the therapist in that it gives the therapy a specific direction, and allows a progressive evaluation of the results achieved; (2) for the patient, defining the goals of therapy is a positive suggestion, and the discussion of and agreement on the duration and the aims of the treatment can reinforce and enhance the patient's willingness to cooperate and commitment to a successful outcome. The patient therefore feels actively involved and in control of the therapeutic process. Moreover, in agreeing on the goals to be reached, the therapist is, in fact, signaling a message to the patient: "I believe you are fully capable of reaching this goal" or "I believe that you will manage to solve your problems." This type of message greatly encourages change and generally motivates the patient to cooperate.

Rosenthal (1966), in his famous experiments, demonstrated the influence of experimenters on the experiments that
they conduct — or, rather, how experimenters influence, through
their expectations, the behavior and efficiency of the experimental objects, be they mice or human beings. Positive expectation
on the part of the experimenter can greatly improve a subject's
performance. The same holds for hypnotherapy: if the hypnotherapist expresses certainty that the subject will go into a trance,
the subject, in fact, will do so.

Finally, in agreeing on the goals of therapy and in plan-
ning to achieve them, it is most important that the therapist
not exert too much pressure and thereby provoke anxiety in the
patient, but rather engage the patient in a gradual progression
of preliminary smaller goals. The patient must not feel forced
to change, but instead should see the treatment as systematic
and thorough, with concrete aims. If the patient feels rushed,
the risk is great that the treatment will go awry. It has in fact
been shown that, paradoxically, encouraging patients to take
their time and go slowly often brings about a change more readily, while attempting to hurry the process along slows down
change by reinforcing the patient's resistance. The person may
even become too intimidated to continue the treatment.

Identifying the Perceptive-Reactive
System Maintaining the Problem

With the first three phases of treatment completed, the therapist must study the patient's situation carefully to determine
the key aspects that sustain the problem. Looked at another way,
the therapist must determine the best strategy to bring about
change. Thus, over and above clarifying the problem, the therapist must also understand how it is maintained and on which
of the factors to act to ensure success.

Clinical experience has shown that, ironically, it is often
the patient's very attempts to solve the problem that, in fact,
maintain it. The attempted solution becomes the true problem.
As in the old joke, recounted earlier, about the drunk searching for his key, the thing that makes the whole situation problematical is not his having lost the key in the first place; this is

not a pathological act, but rather the drunk's attempted solution —
looking for the key under the streetlamp, knowing full well that
he had not lost the key there. His insistence on searching in
the wrong place is the problem. Often patients' attempted solutions become "generalized" and transferred to other situations,
which then, too, become problematical. In these cases, in order
to bring about change, the therapist must intervene at the level
of these attempted solutions, singling out the most fundamental self-reinforcing pattern for direct therapeutic intervention.

At this stage of therapy, the therapist should also carefully evaluate the influence a patient's social interactions may
have on attempted solutions. The therapist may deem it necessary to intervene directly in these interpersonal relationships,
as well as in the attempted solutions, or maybe to concentrate
solely on the reorganization of that relationship system, given
that the attempted solutions will be influenced in turn by the
change in the relationship system as a whole.

The therapist must judge each case individually, decid-
ing whether it would be more effective to intervene at the level
of the dysfunctional perceptive-reactive system of the individual, inducing a chain reaction that can affect interpersonal relationships, or whether it would be preferable to extend the therapy to include more subjects and tackle the problem at the level
of the patient's family relationships, where changes may in turn
alter the perceptive-reactive system of the identified patient.

As pointed out earlier, the therapist needs to decide which
type of relationship (the patient's relationship with self, with
others, or with the world) provides the best starting point for
therapeutic intervention. At this point the appropriate treatment,
indirectly systemic or directly systemic, should be chosen. To
reiterate a key point: instead of investigating presumed intrapsychic factors or presumed past trauma, the therapist is interested in the patient's concrete actions in the here and now
and in the interpersonal and social reactions to these actions.
Clearly, a person's actions are influenced mainly by emotions
and conceptions of reality, but we believe, as we have already
stated, that these, too, only change as a result of concrete experience. Thus, when determining what it is that maintains the

problem, and when applying the strategies for change, it must be remembered that therapy must induce a concrete experience of change. If therapists have correctly followed the phases of treatment to this stage, they should now be in a position both to identify the most effective interventions and to improvise and apply the appropriate strategies.

Therapy Programming and Strategies of Change

Before we consider specific therapeutic procedures, we need to state our belief that it is not legitimate to examine therapeutic strategies out of the context — the particular case — in which they have been developed and used. This is because patient-therapist communication and interaction also contribute to change. The simple fact that patient and therapist communicate at all can sometimes produce therapeutic effects.

In that the process of therapy itself is a therapeutic strategy, our distinction between processes and procedures is a purely linguistic one; in reality these two components of the therapeutic process are indivisible.

The most effective strategies are based on the fundamental axiom of the strategic approach, namely, that "it is the therapy that must adapt itself to the patient, not the patient to the therapy." With this in mind, in preparing an approach, the therapist will use strategies that have previously been effective in similar cases, but will choose or improvise procedures for every individual case. For example, the same general strategy may have to be applied in radically different ways depending on specific social and cultural factors and the personality traits of the patient.

As we have said previously, the therapist must learn the patient's language and representational system in order to present interventions in a way that the patient can readily accept. Thus, a particular form of therapy will never be precisely the same for all patients, but will be modified according to the particular perceptive and communication styles of each individual. In addition, if a strategy proves ineffective, it must be rapidly replaced or supplemented by others.

At this early stage of treatment it is also quite useful to bear in mind that change is much more likely to come about as a result of insisting on apparently minor or even trivial issues and on seemingly unimportant details. In this way patients will not have the impression that excessive demands are made on their capacities and resources, and this, too, is likely to decrease resistance to change. In effect, such seemingly minor and indirect interventions may have far greater effects than imagined.

Such small changes in a system's functioning may set off a chain reaction that will, in the end, restore the system's balance. Thus even seemingly banal or insignificant changes may have great power and should be made full use of in therapy. When, through a gradual progression of small-scale changes, the therapist has brought a person to the point of modifying dysfunctional actions and "images of the world," the therapy has achieved its goal.

Finally, before going on to describe the therapeutic procedures in detail, it is essential to realize that their effectiveness depends not purely and simply on their specific validity for particular symptoms or problems, but above all on the personal influence and charisma of the therapist — a factor that we hold to be a principal determinant of success and failure. The effectiveness of a strategy depends heavily on the suggestive framework within which it is presented to the patient: presented "correctly" it can lead to full (and often involuntary) therapeutic cooperation and thus to a willingness to change.

In order to create this framework of suggestions, the therapist has to learn to utilize what we referred to at the beginning of this book as "injunctive language" (after Brown) and "performative speech acts" (after Austin). This type of therapeutic communication, of which Erickson's hypnotic techniques have been the best examples to date, is fundamental to strategic therapy. It is what we term *hypnotherapy without trance*. In using it, the therapist adopts procedures similar to hypnotic suggestions to bring about change. The most recurrent therapeutic procedures utilized in this approach can be divided into two types: actions and therapeutic communication, and behavioral prescriptions.

Actions and Therapeutic Communication

Learning to Speak the Patient's Language. The first thing the therapist attempts to do is to learn to use the patient's language. This key communication technique derives from Ericksonian hypnotherapy, at least as far as its application in psychotherapy is concerned. Erickson employed communication methods that he had used in trance induction as therapeutic language. In fact, in trance induction, he imitated the patient's perceptive and communicative style, slowly and gradually taking control, until finally persuading the patient to let go and fall into a trance.

Bandler and Grinder (1975b) defined this communication strategy as the "tracing technique." They had studied Erickson's communication techniques and found that in his first encounters with patients he adopted their own style of language and their own personal concepts of reality. Furthermore, he even imitated the patients' forms of nonverbal communication in order to put them completely at their ease, which enabled him to gradually influence them with his suggestions and prescriptions.

But it was not Erickson who first discovered the effectiveness of this persuasion technique; it had been an essential component of classical rhetoric for more than two thousand years. Aristotle, for example, in his *Retorica ad Alexandrum,* said, as did the Sophists, that if you want to persuade someone you must use his own arguments. Moreover, experimental psychology has repeatedly shown that human beings are attracted to, and influenced by, things that are familiar to them or similar to themselves. This knowledge is utilized in tangible and often far from noble ways by professionals of mass persuasion.

For many years the social psychologist Roberto Cialdini has been studying strategies of persuasion, and in one of his studies of the selling techniques employed by insurance agents he found that clients tend to sign the contract more readily if the agent resembles them in some way: age, religion, ideas, language, and the like (Cialdini, 1984). Clients do not realize that salespeople are trained to mimic their language and agree with their views in order to find those points of interpersonal contact that are useful in getting the client to sign on the dotted line. Cialdini also found positive results in his research into the use of these persuasion techniques in winning a person's approval, and, of course, the success of many advertising campaigns is due to the fact that they reflect the life-style and day-to-day language of the target population.

The wealth of such data shows clearly how important it is to adopt communicative techniques that allow the therapist to influence the patient as rapidly as possible. Despite the fact that patients ask for help in changing their problems, they usually, albeit unknowingly, resist change. This resistance can be lessened by using this style of communication. In order to be effective, however, it must be carried out in as natural a way as possible and in no way appear artificial; otherwise, it can have the opposite effect. If the patient feels mocked or ridiculed, resistance will increase.

Careful training in communication is essential for success. This training is not dissimilar to that of actors in that therapists have to learn to adapt their own communicative style and repertory of expressions to the broad spectrum of possible clinical situations. This adaptation, or shall we say "performance," must be as natural as possible if it is to be convincing. Therapists in training should have the opportunity to participate in a wide variety of simulated sessions, to have sessions video-recorded, and thus to monitor their own progress.

We believe that preparation in communicative facility is excellent for promoting mental agility. By learning to adapt their language to various situations, contexts, and personal styles, therapists also learn to continually shift their perspectives on reality, which is essential if they are to be able to solve the great diversity of human problems they will be presented with.

Reframing. Reframing is one of the more subtle techniques of persuasion. It does not change a person's *perception* of reality, but the *meaning* it has for him: this is because by putting the same "fact" into a different context of meaning and so looking at it from a different perspective, its value changes radically. As we have said many times, reality is determined by a person's worldview: if that perspective changes, "reality" changes, too.

Let us take a historical example. During the fifteenth century the heads of the Catholic Church were confronted by the problem of a pagan water cult, which was being practiced in Italy. The local people believed that several of their freshwater springs had supernatural powers. (See Dini, 1980, for explication of the ancient traditions underlying such cults.) The ecclesiastical authorities intervened, trying to stamp out the cult by harshly reprimanding its followers and destroying their shrines. In 1425 Saint Bernard of Siena had soldiers destroy a pagan temple after all his preachings against the cult had been in vain. But even this did not succeed.

At this point, the saint and other churchmen found the solution to the problem, perhaps by remembering what Saint Gregory the Great had done a century before them. They built churches on the sites of the ruined pagan temples and consecrated them to the Virgin Mary, saying that the waters were indeed sacred owing to her presence. In effect, they had reframed popular beliefs in such a way that the cult was no longer at odds with the Church, and the people were therefore free to continue in their conviction that the springs were sacred.

Let us analyze this strategy. In a situation where preaching and violent intervention had been to no avail, a strategic move achieved the desired effect — a move that was in keeping with the popular beliefs but that added one important variable which changed the perceptual perspective of the cult and succeeded in changing it from pagan to Christian. A clinical example of such a move would be the reframing of a phobic person's perception of help. (This approach is described in detail in Chapter Five.) Patients are told that they definitely need, and, in fact, cannot do without the help of other people. But the therapist intimates, by means of double messages, that such help could aggravate their symptoms. In practice, the therapist redirects the fear that has led the patients to ask for help, and thereby stops the help-seeking behavior.

Reframing can be achieved either purely verbally or by certain actions that lead persons to change their view of reality, just as reframing effects can be produced by means of behavioral prescriptions, which will be examined later. Reframing can vary in complexity, going from a simple cognitive redefinition of an idea or behavior pattern to the use of metaphors and evocative suggestions, and even to complicated paradoxical reframings.

In a general sense, all the therapeutic strategies cited here can be considered reframings in that all are ultimately geared toward changing the patient's behavior and point of view. There are those who maintain that verbal reframing by means of dialogue is the key method employed by all forms of psychotherapy (Simon, Stierlin, and Wynne, 1965, p. 286), changing the "mental map" of a patient being the factor common to all forms of psychotherapy. As far as we are concerned, reframing has nothing to do with the job of attributing meaning to emotions. This persuasive strategy works on the perceptive structure on which the subjective interpretations and behavior are based, rather than directly or mainly on the semantic aspects of reality.

At the semantic level, the strategic therapist offers neither reassurance nor confirmation of the meaning of things, but, on the contrary, raises doubts that break the patient's habitual perceptive-reactive rigidity, creating chinks in the patient's cognitive and behavioral armor. Newton Da Costa, a logician at the University of São Paulo, in Brazil, has shown how the raising of doubt regarding the logical rational explanation is particularly effective in unhinging rigid mental structures. Da Costa maintains that in convincing persons to change their opinions it is much more effective to plant doubts about the logic of their reasoning than to demonstrate fully and rationally the incorrectness or inadequacy of their ideas or behavior (personal communication, May 1989).

Doubt can be likened to a woodworm that gets inside a piece of wood and devours it from the inside. Doubt grows by devouring the preexisting logic that surrounds it. Doubt mobilizes the system's entropy, starting a slow but devastating chain reaction, which can lead to changes in the whole system. Therefore, we believe, along with Simon, Stierlin, and Wynne (1985), that reframing a person's "mental map" is the goal of all psychotherapy, but reframing in the strategic approach is completely different from the pursuit of "insight" typical of other therapeutic approaches.

Moreover, the art of reframing as a technique of persuasion

is certainly not a new discovery and does not even have its origins in the therapeutic field; it, too, was a commonly used intervention in classical rhetoric, above all by the Sophists — renowned masters of the verbal art of persuasion. Returning to more recent times, however, social psychology research has shown that a person's perceptions and reactions can be changed, not by directly altering the rational meaning attributed to things, but instead by using reframing techniques.

Perhaps the best experimental demonstration of the enormous power that certain suggestions have to induce change is supplied by Langer, a psychologist at the University of California. Standing in a line of people waiting to use a photocopier in the library, a female student asked if she might go ahead of the others, and, depending on the exact wording of her request, got very different reactions from the other students. When she said, "Excuse me. I've got five pages. May I use the photocopier because I'm in a real hurry?" 95 percent of the students let her go ahead. By contrast, only 60 percent consented when she said, "Excuse me, I've got five pages. May I use the photocopier?" At first glance, it seems that the added explanation "because I'm in a hurry" was all-important. But a third version of the request showed that this was not exactly the case. Here, "because" was included, but nothing else was added: "Excuse me, I've got five pages. Can I use the photocopier because I've got to make the copies?" Ninety-three percent of the people asked agreed, even though they were given no additional information about the request, which might have prompted their acquiescence. Just as the "chip, chip" of the turkey chick triggers an automatic reaction from its mother, even when the "chick" is simply a stuffed imitation, so the word *because* triggered automatic agreement in Langer's subjects, even when no reason was actually given (Cialdini, 1984).

This experiment shows how a person's reactions to a situation can be modified if the situation is reframed, not necessarily in a logical or rational way. It also shows the power of certain suggestive forms of communication to lessen resistance and confuse logical-rational convictions. Thus reframing is not a direct means of attributing meaning, but a way of softening

a person's rigid logic. It opens new horizons and possibilities
for changing the seeming immutability of a person's mindset.

When the therapist restructures a patient's reality, im-
itating the latter's ways of interpreting the environment, the therapist must lead the patient to see things from different points
of view. Suggestion, elements of classical rhetoric, and logical
paradoxes can be utilized, all of which, if used correctly, can
alter a person's perception of reality, if only for a moment.

Avoiding Negative Formulations. The third strategy of
therapeutic communication is directly connected to the first two;
in fact, one could say that it punctuates them. Clinical practice
has shown that negative formulations regarding a person's behavior or ideas are perceived as blame and only provoke resistance. In hypnosis, negative formulations have a similar effect
and, therefore, the hypnotherapist tends to rephrase all negative ideas into positive statements. Instead of criticizing a patient's behavior, even when it is clearly dysfunctional, it is far
more productive to go along with the patient, making him or
her feel at ease, and then to offer suggestions as to how to change
the behavior.

For example, faced with two overprotective parents who,
by their excessive concerns, have made their son insecure and
psychologically fragile, the therapist might compliment them on
having dealt so well with a difficult child, and on all the sacri-
fices they have made in order to protect him from possible dangers
in the outside world. The therapist might say, "And, seeing that
you have done such a good job so far, I'm sure you will manage
admirably to do even better now, in getting him to assume his
responsibilities." At this point the therapist would prescribe radically different actions and behavior for the parents. In this way,
instead of blaming the parents for the mistakes they have made
in bringing up their child and for their suffocating overprotec-
tion, and instead of saying to them "don't do this, don't do that,
you've done this wrong and that wrong," the therapist makes use
of the parents' capacity to intervene, reframing it positively and
giving a direct prescription as to the correct and functional parental behavior that will resolve the problem.

This example combines three different techniques: avoidance of negative formulations, reframing, and prescription. Such techniques generally promote participation and cooperation, even in rigidly difficult patients, and circumvent any negative reactions that blaming the patient might cause. Patients show that they know their actions are dysfunctional by asking for help; there is no need for the therapist to emphasize this.

Use of Paradox and of Paradoxical Communication Patterns. A logical paradox is a statement that is both true and false, correct and incorrect. The classical example is that of the Cretan Epimenides, who said, "All Cretans are liars." Thus the logic trap is constructed, whether true or false, correct or incorrect. In interpersonal communication, such a paradox occurs when there are two logically inconsistent messages within the same communication. The receiver of the message is in the same predicament as anyone wishing to decide whether Epimenides is telling the truth.

We maintain that the use of paradox is a keystone in therapy, often extraordinarily effective in rigid perceptive-reactive situations and circular patterns of self-reinforcing behavior. For this reason, this therapeutic procedure plays a fundamental role in the strategic approach. Paradox unhinges the Aristotelian logic of "true and false" and the Manichean world of opposites (black/white, beautiful/ugly, correct/incorrect) used as categories to describe reality. As far as the philosophy of knowledge is concerned, logical paradox has undermined every attempt to imprison reality within a descriptive and interpretive system of absolute logic.

Applied to the specific therapeutic context, paradox can break the vicious circle of repetitive behavior that constitutes an "attempted solution"—the self-reinforcing behavior pattern from which the patient cannot, or is unwilling to, extricate himself. Paradox undermines the patient's preexisting system of perceptions and reactions regarding reality.

Historically speaking, paradox first entered therapy as a therapeutic strategy under the auspices of Viktor Frankl's "paradoxical intention" (1960). But it was really Bateson, Jackson,

Haley, and Weakland (1956) who first systematically formulated paradox for use in solving problems. They showed that paradox is a basic constituent of mental problems and can be used effectively in their resolution. In other words, they applied the age-old medical dictum "similia similibus curantur" (like is cured by like).

Paradox appears in various formulations in therapy — from paradoxical prescriptions to paradoxical actions and communications. We believe the following examples explain better than any formal analysis can how therapeutic paradoxes work. The first example is of a person, who in classical psychiatric terminology would be considered an "obsessive-hypochondriac," convinced that she is suffering from a serious, incurable disease. Despite conventional medical evidence to the contrary, she persists in this observation and interprets every bodily change that may be a little out of the ordinary as being a symptom of her mysterious illness. She is terrified and seeks reassurance and help from everyone around her, and in particular from her therapist. The following is the transcript of a brief conversation with this patient:

Patient: Doctor, I'm exhausted. I feel so ill! I'm so scared! There's something malignant inside me, I can feel it growing. I'm going to die soon! Nobody believes that I'm seriously ill. I sweat all the time, and I can feel my heart beating so fast. And then, you know, as I told my husband, I feel as if there is a curse on me. You won't believe these things, but it's true. Nobody believes me, but it's eating away my insides.

Therapist: Hmmm. (*Looking serious and pensive*) I really do believe you are seriously ill. In fact, I'm sure that your disease is quite rare. You know there are "curses" and "curses," and it looks as though you've been cursed. (*Brief pause*)

Yes, I really do feel that you will become very ill, and get worse and worse. In fact, looking at you now, it seems that you're getting worse right here in front of me. You feel ill, right? You look to me as if you are going to feel really bad soon. (*Faint smile*)

Patient: But doctor, what are you saying, that I'm going to die? So, it's really true, then. I *am* seriously ill. But, doctor, why haven't all those medical tests I've had done shown anything wrong with me? But are you really sure of what you're saying, that I am ill and that you can really see that someone *has* put a curse on me?

Therapist: But, of course. *(Slight smile)*

Patient: But, doctor, you're making fun of me. I hardly feel ill at all now. In fact, talking to you, I've stopped sweating and I feel much calmer. But, tell me, doctor, how is it that at the age of forty our brains play such tricks on us?

This example shows how, in situations in which rational logic has no effect, paradox can be useful in breaking the repetitive mechanism inherent in obsessions.

Patients are usually worried and surprised when they hear that their terrors are justified. Then, it is they themselves who start to reassure the therapist as to their state of health, saying that the medical tests found nothing wrong. In a few cases, they will smile when they understand the "kind trick" the therapist has been playing. But the important thing is that the obsessive mechanism of distorted perceptions and reactions has been broken, and their point of view and actions regarding the problem can both begin to change. This example is a good illustration of the logic on which paradoxical intervention is based, and how it is particularly well suited to tackling compulsive acts.

Using this technique, a therapist can create a paradox that renders a symptom voluntary rather than out of the patient's control, but in order to be a symptom, in the strict sense of the word, the problem must be involuntary. From the moment that it becomes voluntary, the symptom completely loses its symptomatic quality. When confronted by such rigid obsessive behavior, rather than analyzing and criticizing, the therapist causes it to escalate to a point where it eliminates itself. The mechanism is the same as that involved in the prescription of the symptom: the destructive capacities of paradox are set in action, and the patient's distorted perceptions are deliberately encouraged. Just as a deliberate attempt to be happy when you are depressed only makes you feel worse, and consciously trying to go to sleep only keeps you awake, leading the patient to persist intentionally in those distorted and seemingly uncontrollable mental processes causes them to lose their essential spontaneity and symptomatic status and they disappear.

Another example of the use of paradox illustrates a slightly different kind of paradoxical action and communication, but reveals the same power of bringing about change. It has to do with those interpersonal situations in which an action and/or an unexpected paradoxical message (a message that could not be foreseen from the usual run of events) turns the situations upside down. The message appears to be neither true nor false and is seemingly at odds with the whole situation, motivating the receiver to make a sudden change in behavior. The enormous effectiveness of such interpersonal communication devices is well illustrated by a strange event that took place in Austria at the end of the 1920s. It received considerable newspaper coverage by virtue of the peculiarities of the case. A young man wishing to commit suicide threw himself off a bridge into the Danube River. A policeman drawn to the scene by the shouts of the onlookers put his rifle to his shoulder and, aiming it at the young man in the water, shouted, "Get out, or I'll shoot!," at which point the young man came meekly out of the water, relinquishing his suicide attempt. In effect, the policeman's action put the youth in a paradoxical situation. The forcible reframing of his reality led him to radical changes in his behavior and his thought processes. In clinical practice, as in life in general, such paradoxical experiences, apparently illogical and completely unforeseen by the patient, rapidly produce that jump in logic, indispensable for changing a situation.

From these examples it is clear how effective paradoxes can be in unhinging the rigid, obsessive situations that many patients create for themselves. The use of paradoxes, albeit in a multitude of different formats, is particularly effective in the early phase of strategic therapy, when the therapist has to break the self-reinforcing system of perceptions, actions, and reactions that is maintaining the patient's problem.

The Utilization of Resistance. The utilization of resistance, one of the most refined techniques derived from the paradox, is of great value in therapy. As far as resistance is concerned, we believe, contrary to classical psychoanalytical thinking, that the energy invested in resistance can be redirected so that it can be of great assistance in achieving therapeutic goals. I also recommend that resistance itself be paradoxically prescribed and thus manipulated. This is done by creating a therapeutic double bind: the patient's resistance — rigidity toward the therapist — becomes a prescription in itself, and the patient's subsequent reactions constitute the therapeutic progress. In this way, the primary effect of the resistance is eliminated, and its underlying energy is put into the service of change; a prescribed resistance, in fact, ceases to be resistance and becomes compliance. Consider this therapist's response to a difficult and distrustful patient. The therapist says, "Look, there is a strong possibility that we can solve your problem, and there are some specific techniques that we could use. But, looking at the circumstances as they stand at the moment, coupled with your outlook on the situation, I don't believe you will succeed." The patient now finds herself in a paradoxical situation. Her usual reaction (her bottled-up aggression toward the therapist) motivates her to do exactly what the therapist said she was incapable of doing. The patient thus collaborates with the therapist, and her resistance is eliminated.

Students of some martial arts learn to use their opponent's strength to their own advantage by combining the natural force of gravity and a sharpened sense of balance. Similarly, this technique redirects the force of the patient's resistance to promote change. The expert hypnotist uses this strategy in reframing a subject's resistance so that she will let herself go into a deeper trance. For example, if the patient resists going into a trance by moving her fingers or her leg, the hypnotist will say, "Very good, your hand [or leg] is responding, now start to move it faster and faster until you feel tired and really want to rest." Thus, resistance is redefined and its power is directed toward trance induction.

The Use of Metaphor, Anecdotes, and Stories. Other important means of therapeutic communication are the use of metaphor, anecdotes, and story telling in the sense of recounting events involving other people. These strategies allow the therapist to communicate messages, albeit indirectly, by the identification and projection that people often feel regarding characters and situations in fiction. This technique minimizes resistance because patients are not requested to do anything, nor are their opinions or behavior criticized. The message gets through in disguise, in a manner of speaking. Let us consider an obsessive or phobic patient: in order to get across to him just how counterproductive it is to listen incessantly to oneself, thereby increasing one's anxiety to the point of a panic attack, a therapist might tell the story of the centipede which, when it stopped to think how it managed to walk so elegantly with so many legs to move at once, found it could no longer walk at all. The therapist might then get the patient to try the following exercise: "When you leave the room, do what the centipede did: as you walk down the stairs, concentrate on just how difficult it is to keep your balance step after step, putting your foot down in just the right place. Usually, you know, a person starts to stumble and finds he can't walk any farther." This type of tactic is far more effective than giving the patient a scientific explanation. Suggestions are embedded in a story or communicated through metaphors in such a way that the patient is not directly involved, but the evocative power of the story or image counteracts the patient's self-reinforcing conceptions and behaviors.

In strictly linguistic terms, the therapist is making use of the message's "poetic function," that is, the evocative power of these forms of communication (Jakobson, 1963). All of us have felt the effects of a particularly touching poem, a passage in a book, or a film. We have felt that we ourselves were really the protagonists; even knowing full well that it is all pretense, our emotions are touched and we live a real and concrete experience. Again, it was Erickson who led the way in inducing this kind of experience in therapy. He brought to psychotherapy what was already known to hypnotists. Indeed, it is usual for a hypnotist to induce a trance by narrating an evocative story that carries suggestions, usually in the form of metaphor. It does not detract from Erickson's originality to note that the power of this persuasion strategy has been used in a variety of contexts for many centuries.

Anyone who is skeptical about the power of evocative language will find it difficult to dismiss what the famous sociologist David Phillips termed the "Werther Effect" (1974, 1979, 1980). It has a long and interesting history. Goethe's *The Sorrows of Young Werther* recounts the story of a young man who, heartbroken over an ill-fated love affair, commits suicide. Its publication had a shattering effect on the society of the day. Apart from the fame and fortune it earned for Goethe, the book provoked a wave of similar suicides throughout Europe. There were so many in some countries that the authorities banned the book altogether.

Phillips's research looks at how the Werther Effect manifests itself in modern times — how, for example, a front-page suicide story in a newspaper will dramatically increase the number of suicides among readers of that newspaper. Phillips analyzed suicide statistics in the United States from 1947 to 1968, and found that in the two months following a front-page report of a suicide, there were on average fifty-eight more suicides than normal. Furthermore, there were striking similarities between the subsequent suicides and the original one, in particular with regard to age and social class of the victims.

But Phillips did not stop there. He went on to show that the Werther Effect is equally applicable to other events, such as acts of violence and heroism. The only two prerequisites are that the act be publicized and that the receiver either be similar or *feel* similar to the actor in the original report. Phillips's evidence clearly shows the strength of projection and identification mechanisms, and their power to evoke emulative behavior in receivers of the message who see themselves as similar to the protagonist of a moving story.

Given that psychotherapy is primarily aimed at provoking change in a patient's consciousness and behavior, we must not overlook or underestimate the extraordinary power that can be exercised through the narration of stories and anecdotes that fit in well with the patient's problematical reality. They can lead the patient to make tangible changes in behavior patterns, which in turn can lead to change in perceptive and cognitive makeup.

Behavioral Prescriptions. Behavioral prescriptions are directives that a patient is to follow between sessions. They play a fundamental role in strategic therapy. As we have said, in order to change, one has to undergo concrete experiences; behavioral prescriptions make such concrete experiences of change a reality outside the therapeutic setting.

Behavioral prescriptions merit our particular attention because when patients act alone and in their daily routines they can give themselves the best possible demonstration of their ability to change their problem situations. The fact that they do certain things unknowingly, in response to the therapist's "kind tricks," does not change this assertion, because, knowingly or unknowingly, they have still achieved something of which they were previously incapable. Such experiences are the tangible and indisputable proof of the ability to overcome one's difficulties. They clearly open up new perspectives regarding the problem situation; in other words, they break the mechanism of actions and reactions and "attempted solutions" that maintain it. Behavioral prescriptions can be divided into three types: *direct, indirect,* and *paradoxical.*

Direct prescriptions are clear instructions to carry out specific actions. They are aimed at the resolution of the problem or at reaching one of a series of goals on the road to change. This technique is useful for cooperative patients who show little resistance to change. It gives them the key to the resolution of the problem, indicating to them how to act in order to break the mechanism that maintains the problem. Let us consider the case of a man and wife who are continually arguing because, with the best of intentions, each is trying to correct the "bad behavior" of the other. It is easy to see how this simply leads to more and more quarrels. In fact, it becomes a never-ending cycle of actions and reactions.

In such a situation, if just one of the partners becomes more cooperative, it will be sufficient to break the vicious circle of corrections and countercorrections. The therapist need only explain the situation clearly, giving the client the job of breaking the chain, either by not reacting at all to the partner's corrective behavior or by giving the partner the last word.

During the phase immediately following this change in the system that has kept the problem alive, the therapist can use direct prescription to help the patient successfully handle the situations that previously were problematical. To this end, the therapist tells the patient what to do, directly and explicitly, giving a series of step-by-step instructions.

Indirect prescriptions are behavioral injunctions whose real objectives are hidden. The therapist prescribes an action that will produce a different result from the one that was seemingly being specified. This type of prescription utilizes the hypnotic technique of shifting the symptom: usually the patient's attention is drawn to a secondary problem, thereby reducing the intensity of the problem originally presented.

To better explain this technique, let us use the analogy of a magician: the magician draws the audience's attention with some obvious, dramatic movements so that her subtle tricks are not noticed, thus producing a spectacular and seemingly magical effect. For example, if the therapist instructs a phobic patient to carry out an anxiety-provoking and embarrassing exercise every time the symptoms manifest themselves, such as writing down in detail the feelings and thoughts that occur at that moment and bringing them to the session, the patient may return ridden with guilt because he has not done what the therapist required. Strangely, he says (and he cannot explain why), he did not suffer any phobic symptoms during the whole week. Obviously, it was either the embarrassment or the anxiety provoked by the exercise that prevented the symptoms from appearing. In other words, his attention was shifted away from the problem itself onto the exercise he was supposed to carry out. This "kind trick" succeeded in neutralizing the problematical symptoms. But, more important, the patient saw, by means of a concrete experience, that he could control and even eliminate his symptoms. Because they reduce resistance to change by getting the patient to do something without realizing that he is doing it, these interventions play a fundamental role in the first phase of strategic treatment.

Paradoxical prescriptions are a natural progression from the previously described utilization of paradox in therapy. In the case of a seemingly spontaneous and unsolvable problem, such as repetitive obsessions or other particularly resistant dysfunctional behavior, they can be very effective. The patient finds herself in a paradoxical situation, having to perform voluntarily actions that had previously been involuntary and uncontrollable, and that she had always tried to avoid. In this case, also, the voluntary performance of the symptom eliminates it, as it is no longer spontaneous and uncontrollable.

For example, consider the case of a patient who manifested the nightly ritual of checking over and over again that he had turned off all faucets, lights, and gas switches, and that his shoes were exactly placed in a particular position, before he could go to sleep. The prescriptions given to this patient were as follows: every evening to (a) voluntarily and extremely carefully turn off the lights and the gas switches a specific number of times, using both hands; and (b) to position his shoes just as he had always done, but to point the shoes in the opposite direction. Within two weeks the nightly rituals ceased. Paradoxical prescriptions, like indirect prescriptions, can be very effective in lessening a patient's resistance to change and are thus of great therapeutic value in the early phases of therapy.

In order for prescriptions to be followed and to be effective they need to be very carefully formulated and then presented to the patient almost as hypnotic commands, using the therapeutic communication techniques described above. The use of injunctive or hypnotic language is crucial to their effectiveness in psychotherapy; otherwise, patients rarely carry out the prescriptions they are given, in particular those that are indirect or paradoxical (see Watzlawick, 1978). This may explain why some therapists complain about the ineffectiveness of prescriptive and paradoxical methods.

Prescriptions must be given to the patient in a slow and repetitive manner at the end of the session. This technique is clearly analogous to hypnotic trance induction. We have seen the effectiveness of behavioral prescriptions in producing change in the therapeutic setting, but what about their effectiveness (in other contexts) as instruments of persuasion? One only has to

think of tribal initiation ceremonies that promote social acceptance and that probably go back to the beginnings of humankind.
To conclude, however, it is most important that, after a prescription is carried out, the result be examined in detail and the patient praised for progress thus far. The patient should be made
aware that the problems thought to be insoluble can, in fact,
be overcome in a nonstressful way — and that the patient's achieve-
ments to date demonstrate this. Prescriptions can be formulated
in a variety of ways and may involve very different patterns of
behavior: they can be simple tasks to do at home, complicated
rituals, or even actions that seemingly have nothing to do with
the patient's problem. The important thing is that the therapist
use the maximum inventiveness and imagination to find the key
to unlock the dysfunctional system of actions and reactions in
which the patient is caught.

Termination

The final session in a course of strategic therapy plays an important role: it is the finishing touch, the frame that surrounds
the completed painting. The goal is to consolidate the autonomy of the patient. The therapist does this by giving a résumé
of the entire course of therapy, explaining in detail the therapeutic process, the strategies used, and the often strange techniques (indirect injunctions, suggestions, paradoxical prescriptions) employed. This final exposé is crucial if the patient is to
gain autonomy, to know that the "psychic and behavioral" reality
has changed, thanks to systematic and scientific intervention,
and not to some strange form of magic. Above all, it emphasizes how the person tenaciously but unsuccessfully sought the
solution of the problem, and that now, having completed this
difficult task, the patient is capable of independently dealing with
any future problems.

    At every stage of the treatment, the therapist tries to avoid
creating dependency on the part of the patient. After every small
change, the patient must be praised for the hard work and efforts
expended in solving the problem. Moreover, right from the beginning, brief therapy induces the patient to assume responsi-

bility for personal actions and, indeed, for the progress of the therapy itself. The therapist's management of the situation and personal influence on the patient are both geared to instill in the patient the capacity to solve the problem as quickly as possible.

Finally, it should be emphasized that, during therapy, it is the qualities and characteristics that already existed within the patient that have been activated and that, after therapy, the patient recognizes and is able to use. Nothing has been added that was not within before. The patient has learned to perceive reality differently and to act accordingly.

Chapter 5

Models for Treating
Phobic and Obsessive Disorders

Learning is acquired not to show it off, but to use it.
—G. C. Lichtenberg, *The Little Book of Consolation*

We believe that therapists can prepare, and have at their disposal, a series of strategies that can be relied on to lead to the resolution of specific types of problems. It is obvious that any such program would always require adaptation to meet the needs and circumstances of each person with whom the therapist works.

In this chapter we present specific treatment models that we have devised for phobic problems (panic attacks and agoraphobia) and for problems related to compulsive rituals and obsessive fixations. Our method was to apply the same procedure in several cases, to videotape the sessions, and then to evaluate the work. This methodology permitted progressive adjustment of the aim of the initial hypotheses of therapeutic protocol by enabling us to identify the most efficacious and efficient strategic therapies as well as the most appropriate process—from the "opening moves" to the final "checkmate" of the problem. The two models explained in this chapter are the final results of our research with patients who exhibited phobic and obsessive disorders.

Treatment of Phobic Disorders

Phobic disorders presented by the patients who came to us for treatment can be subdivided into two categories, based on their severity. The first category is represented by severe forms of agoraphobia and panic attacks, the second by less serious forms of the same problems — marked, nevertheless, by strong crises of anxiety and fear.

In order to better clarify the concept of severe forms of agoraphobia and panic attacks, we turn to a psychological problem that can be defined as the "fear of fear." Because of their fear, all patients who manifested this problem abandoned any activity that required a minimum of commitment, responsibility, or personal involvement (work, sports, hobbies, parties, and the like). They were equally incapable of being out alone and of remaining at home alone. Each minor physical stimulus was transformed into a signal of alarm and provoked terror. Each proprioceptive stimulus or bodily sensation was taken to be a symptom of illness and, in turn, provoked panic attacks. The situation was insufferable for the individuals as well as for those close to them (spouses, family, friends, who generally felt compelled to promise never to abandon these patients).

The symptoms exhibited by patients in the second category were less serious. These patients were not incapable of pursuing their usual activities, but did so with considerable effort and at an extremely reduced productivity level. In each of these cases, the patient frequently manifested panic attacks and immobilizing fears that at times were not preceded by any apparent cause. The patients were incapable of doing anything to fight their fears.

Treatment Modalities

In order to make clear the process and the procedure utilized in this type of treatment, we think it helpful to present a summary of the treatment itself. The therapeutic process is subdivided into four characteristic stages by preestablished objectives to be achieved before passing on to the next stage, and by specific strategic interventions for each stage.

Summary of the Treatment

I.   First stage: from the first to the third session
     A.   Objectives:
          1.   obtain trust and collaboration

 2. break down the rigid system of reality perception
 3. demonstrate that change is possible
 B. Strategies:
 1. speaking the language of the patient
 2. reframing of the problem
 3. indirect prescriptions
 4. redefinition of effects and changes
II. Second stage: from the third to the fifth session
 A. Objectives:
 1. strengthening the capacity for change
 2. effective change of the situation
 3. cognitive reframing
 B. Strategies:
 1. paradoxical prescriptions
 2. reframing
 3. go-slow technique
III. Third stage: from the fifth session onward
 A. Objectives:
 1. bring about concrete examples of gradual mastery of the problem
 2. redefinition of the perception of self, others, and the world
 B. Strategies:
 1. direct behavior prescriptions accompanied by specific suggestions
 2. redefinition of the situation after each compliance with the prescription
IV. Fourth stage: the last session
 A. Objectives:
 1. encouragement of personal autonomy
 B. Strategies:
 1. detailed explanation of the type of work done together and of the techniques used
 2. conclusive redefinition of the capacity demonstrated in confronting and resolving the problem (positive suggestions for the future)

First Stage: From the First to the Third Session. The first session represents an extremely important phase in the treatment of phobic patients, as such persons have an urgent need to find a solution to their problem. If they do not immediately have a sense of having found the appropriate help, they drop out of treatment. Therefore, it is essential to begin as soon as possible with specific therapeutic interventions.

After having carefully listened to the description of the problem and agreed on the goals of therapy — and using the technique of "copying" as a means of establishing a functional therapeutic collaboration — we attempt the first therapeutic intervention. This is a reframing of the phobic patient's pattern of interpersonal relations.

Usually, this type of person is receiving massive social support from his or her spouse, relatives, friends, or others. As soon as the patient enters into a crisis and asks for help, these figures offer prompt attention to make the patient feel protected and calm. This type of social support functions as an "attempted solution" that maintains the problem. In other words, instead of helping the patient to overcome phobic fears, the helpers' soothing, protective behaviors feed into the problem and keep it alive — and keep the patient trapped in the inability to cope with fear alone.

The first therapeutic step will, consequently, have to be the disruption of the interpersonal system of maintaining the problem. Our first move, then, is directed toward the patient's perception of this support system and habitual reactions to it. The patient needs to see that the support and help received so far have not and will not change the condition. The patient not only must not count on the support and protection of others but also must not accept such dangerous and damaging help because it can aggravate the problem — even if at the moment it is impossible to do without it.

Continuing in the same tone, we explain how the people around the patient are at this point an integral part of the dysfunctional system and how, being so involved, they can do nothing to change the patient's situation. What their support and help produces is simply the confirmation of the patient's incapacity and dependence on them. This functions in such a subtle manner that the situation can only worsen. Nevertheless, we state that for the moment the patient cannot do without the help of others.

As the reader will have already understood, this first reframing is aimed at redirecting the patient's fear, motivating the patient toward the actions that will rupture the system of interpersonal relations that contributes to the perseverance of the problem. By redefining the support and help of others as something that augments the symptoms, we shift the patient's perspective on relationships with others. The patient now sees their protectiveness not as helpful but as damaging and dangerous. To establish this new perception means to induce fear of being helped, because to be helped means to aggravate symptoms. In practice, then, the strength of the phobic disorder is utilized for the purpose of weakening the dysfunctional network of support.

It is important to emphasize in this reframing that, notwithstanding all that has been said, we maintain that initially the patient cannot do without the help of others. This is a paradoxical injunction that usually expands the willingness of the patient, who will want to demonstrate to the therapist an ability to manage without "help" and will collaborate with the therapist in finding a resolution to the problem.

After this first therapeutic action, which usually occupies most of the session, we go on to the first behavioral prescription to be carried out within the context of daily life, but affirming that for the moment—in the initial phase—the assigned task is only an explorative step that must be followed to the letter in order to allow a better understanding of the situation. This is said so that the patient, in carrying out the task, will avoid examining its effects too closely and thereby inhibit the efficacy of the prescription.

The prescription is presented as follows: "Each time, even if it happens a hundred times a day, that you enter into a crisis, have a moment of panic, or feel your anxiety rising, you will take out this log that I am giving you and you will note everything that happens, scrupulously following the enclosed instructions in every detail. At our next session, you will leave me the pages relative to the week in question and I will study them." The log is a pad of extremely boring forms with about ten columns in which to record the date, place, situation, thoughts, actions, symptoms, and the like. At least five minutes are required to fill out a form each time a crisis occurs.

In all the cases presented here, the effect of the prescription was more or less the same. At the second session the patient had made a start, saying, "Doctor, you must excuse me, I haven't done my assignment. But, oddly, this week I didn't have any crises." Or, "You know, doctor, it's strange, but I felt decisively better. I had some critical moments, but, incredibly—I don't know how to explain it—when I wrote the log, the anxiety and fear left me immediately." What happened? How is it possible to have achieved such change?

The rigid view of reality that constrained the patient to determined dysfunctional responses was ruptured. The counterproductive network of social supports was annulled. The "spell" was broken. The most probable explanation of this phenomenon seems to be the following: the prescribed assignment and the reframing executed during the session constrained the patient against using the usual "attempted solutions," which instead of resolving the problem complicated it (for example, the patient habitually makes a strong effort to seek the help of others or not to think about the crisis experience). The obligation to carefully write out events and thoughts placed the patient in a completely new relationship to the phobic fear; logging in each episode is such an annoying assignment that the phobic patient finds ways of avoiding it. In other words, an annoying task preempts the fear and thus blocks it; here again, therefore, the intensity of the symptom is used for its own elimination.

At the second session, after the patient's report about the preceding week, we move on to a therapeutic action that reinforces the effect of the preceding intervention: the redefinition of the situation. We say, "Therefore, the problem isn't as serious as it seemed if a simple prescription was enough to modify the situation. Your problems are not so impossible or inescapable, and you can really change, as you have demonstrated this week." We insist on this redefinition of the problem for the duration of the session. With this, together with the rupture of the rigid system of dysfunctional reactions, we strengthen the patient's self-confidence. The patient's conscious perception of reality begins to shift from a dysfunctional perspective to a more functional one.

If the response to the initial therapeutic intervention has been adequate, at the end of the second session we move on to the second stage; otherwise, the prescription is maintained for another week and the redefinition is repeated in the third session.

Second Stage: From the Third to the Fifth Session. In the last minutes of the second (or third) session, a new behavior prescription is given: a paradoxical assignment of the "be spontaneous" type: "I see that you have been so successful in the preceding weeks in fighting your problem that I am now going to give you an assignment that will appear even stranger and more absurd than the one you have carried out so far. But, as we have agreed, you must do it. I believe that I have earned a bit of your trust, right? Good. You will need an alarm clock for this exercise, one with an annoying ring. Every day at the same time, which we will now agree upon, you must take this alarm clock and set it to go off in half an hour. Then you must close yourself up in a room of your house, sit in a chair, and force yourself to concentrate on your worst fantasies regarding your problem. You will think of your worst fears until you voluntarily produce a crisis of anxiety and panic. Then you will remain in this state for the rest of the half hour. As soon as the alarm clock sounds, turn it off and discontinue the exercise, stopping these thoughts and sensations, and resuming your usual daily activities."

The possible effects of this paradoxical prescription are of two kinds. The first: "Doctor, I wasn't able to throw myself into the situation. I tried, but it seemed so ridiculous that I wound up laughing." The second: "Doctor, I succeeded so well in doing the assignment that I felt the same sensations that I was feeling before coming to you. I suffered enormously, but fortunately the alarm sounded and it ended." It is noteworthy that most patients experienced no moments of crisis outside the half-hour assignment, and several had only infrequent episodes of anxiety, which were easily controlled.

At the next session, after the patient's report on the effect of the prescription, we take steps to again redefine the situation. In the case of the first type of response to the prescription, the redefinition is as follows: "As you were able to prove to yourself, your problem can be lessened by provoking it voluntarily. It is a paradox, but, you know, at times our minds function more by paradox than by logic. You are learning not to fall into the trap of your disorder and of your 'attempted solutions,' which complicate the problem instead of resolving it." The entire session proceeds along this line. In the case of the second type of response, the redefinition is as follows: "Very well, you are learning to modulate and manage your disorder. Just as it is capable of provoking symptoms, you are able to limit them." And so we continue for the duration of the session.

In both situations, therefore, the patient has concrete experiences of the efficacy of therapy. On the one hand, this leads to an exceptional collaboration, and, on the other, to a progressive, ultimate change in the patient's perception of reality. In addition, we are careful to attribute responsibility for the change to the personal capacities of the patient, presenting the therapist as the strategist who used specific techniques to make capabilities emerge that the person already possessed but did not know how to use. This consideration greatly motivates the patient, who has always considered himself inept (an idea confirmed by the behavior of friends and family). Thus attention is focused on increasing the patient's personal competence and autonomy.

After several weeks, the situation may change radically. In all the cases we have referred to in this section, the gripping and immobilizing symptoms disappeared, but the patients could not yet consider themselves cured. At this point, the therapist needs to reduce euphoria and put the patient on guard about the danger of an excessively rapid cure. The watchword now is "go slow." (For a description of the "go-slow" technique in brief therapy, see Fisch, Weakland, and Segal, 1982.) It is essential that patients slow down and realize that if they step on the accelerator too much they may go off the road and fall back into their problems. The important thing, now, is to consolidate that which has been obtained, and so we move on to the next stage.

Third Stage: From the Fifth Session Onward.
In the third stage, we give direct behavior prescriptions that relate to a progressive sequence of anxiety-producing situations to which the patient is gradually exposed. This is analogous to what is done in systematic behavior desensitization, but, in this case, to each direct behavior prescription we add a suggestion that helps the person to carry out the anxiety-laden assignment.

For example, a thirty-three-year-old woman who chose driving a car as her first direct assignment was asked to carefully describe a panic episode that had occurred while she was driving and which she remembered quite vividly. She related that driving on a country road near Arezzo she had had such an attack of fear that she had to stop and ask for help. She was assisted by another driver, who accompanied her to the nearest emergency room. After that episode, it became impossible for her to drive on city streets.

Our prescription was the following: "That's all right. I believe that if you follow my instructions to the letter, after all that you have managed to do in the past few weeks, you will certainly be able to meet this first test. You must, as usual, do exactly what I ask. Tomorrow, after lunch, go to the garage, start the car, and drive along the same road you were on when you had the panic attack. However, instead of going in the same direction, this time go in the opposite direction [first suggestion]. But let me think for a moment. . . . Are you sure that about midway on the road there is a brief detour that leads to that fruit stand where they sell apples that are grown out there? Since I am crazy about apples, you will take that detour and buy me the largest and sweetest apple that you can find at that stand. You will then immediately bring it to me here at my office. I will be busy and will not be able to spend time with you, so ring my doorbell and just give me the apple. Then we will see each other again at our next appointment [second suggestion]."

The next day, the woman rang my bell. She was radiant

and smiling, and handed me an enormous apple. At the next appointment, a week later, she said that each afternoon of the preceding week she had gone for a drive, venturing farther and farther without the least fear, and really enjoying herself very much.

In practice, the patient was given an anxiety-laden prescription situated between two suggestions, the first relative to the assignment itself, the second relative to a different assignment that depended on the first for its execution. The attention of the patient was to be focused on the second assignment and not on the first, the anxiety-laden task. Once both were carried out, the patient reported that she had really overcome her fear. She understood the trick, but had also demonstrated to herself, by an undeniably concrete action, the possibility of overcoming her difficulties.

In contrast to the classical behavior desensitization, which often fails because the patient refuses to execute the direct behavior prescriptions, we even managed to obtain — by means of a "beneficial confusion" — the execution of prescriptions which, if presented by themselves, would fail. Just as jugglers and magicians shift the attention of the observer while they execute their tricks, the anxiety is outwitted in this kind of detour.

In the third stage, the treatment continued in the form of direct behavior prescriptions, each relative to the agreed-upon list of anxiety-laden situations. It is important to remember that after each prescription, as in the initial phases of the therapy, steps were taken to redefine the patient's capacities, as demonstrated in her overcoming a situation that would, initially, have thrown her into crisis. In addition, little by little, the suggestions that accompanied the prescriptions were lessened, to leave only the prescriptions themselves.

Proceeding in this way, a point is usually reached at which the patient affirms a newfound ability to confront — without any problems whatsoever — situations that would previously have been anxiety-laden. That is the moment to move on to the last phase of treatment.

Fourth Stage: Last Session. The last meeting, as already explained, is geared toward consolidating the personal autonomy of the patient. Toward this end, we proceed to a detailed recapitulation and explanation of the therapeutic process undertaken and the strategies utilized, carefully explaining their function, and underscoring the fact that the change that occurred was owing to the patient's personal abilities. The therapist had only activated these already-present personal capabilities and did not (could not) add anything to the process.

On this basis, therapy concludes with the statement that the patient has learned to use his or her own personal gifts and thus has no further need for help.

Efficacy and Effectiveness of the Treatment

The procedure explained above was applied to forty-one patients, who exhibited all the symptoms of phobic disturbances.

The sample consisted of twenty-four women and seventeen men, of a median age of thirty-one, eighteen years being the age of the youngest patient and seventy-one the age of the oldest. Their social standings were varied, as were their occupations, which ranged from teacher, professional, and doctor, to worker, housewife, and student. We can, consequently, claim that the sample was composed of quite diverse personalities, comparable only with respect to their phobias, and also that the study was statistically significant given the number of cases treated. (Note that the efficacy and effectiveness of strategic therapy are explained at length in Chapter Seven. In this chapter we will limit our discussion to evaluation of the cases described here.)

Efficacy. The efficacy of treatment in the cases just described was evaluated on the basis of (a) the final outcome of the therapy, and (b) whether the results were maintained over time or, on the contrary, the symptoms returned or other new symptoms developed in their place.

On the basis of these methodological criteria, the results of the treatment were as follows:

> Thirty-two cases were completely resolved: there was complete resolution of the problem and no relapses occurred within a year.

Seven cases were much improved: there was complete remission of symptoms at the end of therapy, but in follow-up the clients reported sporadic and slight anxiety crises, which were quickly controlled.

Two cases showed little improvement: there was partial symptom reduction at the end of treatment, but in follow-up the clients reported having had frequent moments of anxiety and panic. However, such critical moments were defined by the patients as less strong than those before therapy.

No case remained unchanged.

No case worsened.

This evidence means that the treatment resulted in complete success in 78 percent of the cases; successful treatment with light relapses over time occurred in 17 percent of the cases; and little success was achieved in 5 percent of the cases, either during or following treatment (see Table 5.1).

Table 5.1. Efficacy of Treatment of Phobic Disorders.

Case Outcome	Cases	
	N	%
Resolved	32	78
Much improved	7	17
Little improved	2	5
Unchanged	-	-
Worsened	-	-
Total	41	100

Effectiveness. The median duration of therapy was 15.6 sessions, with a minimum of 6 sessions and a maximum of 34 sessions. To better evaluate the efficiency of therapy, we have subdivided the treatment with a positive outcome — cases resolved or considerably improved — into four groups: therapy lasting from 6 to 10 sessions, from 11 to 20 sessions, from 21 to 30 sessions, and from 31 to 34 sessions. From this breakdown of the data we see that close to 80 percent of the cases were treated in fewer than 20 sessions (see Table 5.2).

Table 5.2. Effectiveness of Treatment of Phobic Disorders.

Total Number of Sessions	Cases Resolved or Much Improved	
	N	%
6–10	9	23
11–20	22	57
21–30	6	15
31–34	2	5

Note: Median duration of treatment = 15.6 sessions.

Reflections on the Results

The data relative to the results obtained from the application of our therapeutic model for phobic disorders amply demonstrate its efficacy. In 95 percent of the cases, patients achieved remission of their symptoms by the end of treatment, although in seven of these, patients later experienced light but controllable relapses. It is noteworthy that only 5 percent obtained scant results and that no case grew worse or remained entirely unchanged after treatment.

In conclusion, the most significant fact to emerge from this analysis of the results is the surprising efficiency of this kind of treatment. Close to 80 percent of the cases were treated in fewer than twenty sessions, and in only four to five months. If we compare such a time commitment with the usual psychotherapeutic timeframe, it is clear that this treatment protocol is capable of producing effective results in brief periods of time.

The Treatment of Obsessive Disorders

Patients in the group described in this section all exhibited fairly severe forms of obsession and compulsive actions. These patients suffered from strong fixations and mania and were obsessed with the need to repeat a variety of "rituals" or, in some cases, to repeat an action and to constantly verify its correctness. Their thoughts were always concentrated on keeping their fixations out of their minds, but the more they were determined not to do or think certain things, the more driven they were to repetitions and rituals, and to ruminating in an ever more contorted manner.

Some specific examples will give a better idea of the problems these patients exhibited. A young accountant, obsessively fearful of making mistakes, checked and rechecked a growing number of invoices and other materials until, exhausted, he eventually collapsed and had to take a temporary leave of absence. A young man obsessed and distressed by the idea that he might be homosexual subjected himself to daily marathons of pornographic films and magazines in order to measure and verify his level of response to feminine or masculine subjects. A woman, persecuted by the conviction that she had run into a pedestrian, was compelled to return to the site of the supposed "crime" with another person who would confirm that what she believed was not true. A husband convinced that his wife was betraying him managed to find contorted confirmation of this in even the most unbelievable circumstances and followed his wife wherever she went, watching her every move. A young woman, before going to bed, would check all faucets, doors, and windows in her house several times. During the night she would awaken and repeat the entire ritual.

In all these cases, the situation had become insufferable. Many of the patients were unable to work. Each patient's obsessions had become increasingly pervasive, diminishing a bit after the performance of certain compulsive actions, but forcefully returning to center stage after very little time.

Summary of the Treatment

   I.   First stage: from the first to the third session
        A.   Objectives:
            1.   obtain trust and collaboration
            2.   break the obsessive succession of thoughts and actions
            3.   produce an initial small concrete change
        B.   Strategies:
            1.   support the patient's obsessions
            2.   paradoxical reframing and confusion technique

    3. symptom prescription
    4. use of anecdotes and stories
II. Second stage: from the fourth to the sixth session
     A. Objectives:
         1. strengthening of the initial small concrete change
         2. shift of attention from self to others
         3. further progress toward change
     B. Strategies:
         1. go-slow paradox
         2. paradoxical anticipation of relapse
         3. prescription of the "anthropologist"
III. Third stage: from the sixth session onward
 A. Objectives:
         1. progressive consolidation of the capacity not to slide back into the obsessions
         2. redefinition of the perception of self, others, and the world
     B. Strategies:
         1. redefinition of the actual situation
         2. prescription of the "magic formula"
IV. Fourth stage: the final session
     A. Objectives:
         1. definitive consolidation of the patient's capacity for personal autonomy
     B. Strategies:
         1. detailed explanation of the type of work done
         2. conclusive redefinition of the courage and capacity demonstrated by the patient

First Stage: From the First to the Third Session. The first meeting with the patient was, as usual, geared toward the creation of an atmosphere of interpersonal contact and acceptance. To this end, with obsessive patients more so than with others, it is essential to support and accept their fixations and their contorted thinking patterns. Otherwise, a counterproductive relationship is immediately established. The therapist who seeks to convince patients of the absurdity of their convictions in order to alter their behavior sets into motion a process based on the notion of "common sense," which cannot effect any change in the patients because they are left with the impression of not having been understood.

On the contrary, the more productive point of departure for the treatment of such patients is based on the logical paradox established in the first session: to demonstrate active acceptance of their odd fixations, suggesting that their absurd convictions may be reasonable, and implying that they may even serve a useful purpose.

In the final part of the first session we proceeded to an elaborate, tortuous, pedantic, and unclear reframing of the complaint, quoting from the patient's previous accounts, stating that very often such disorders can play an important — even determinant — role. They are defined, we said, as an additional gift, reserved for especially attentive, sensitive humans. We ended the session with the suggestion that the patient reflect on this possibility in the course of the following week.

In this way we redefined the symptom, implying that it could have a positive function and that this aspect should be investigated. This amounted to a further complication of the already intricate network of the patient's thoughts, leading the person to a paradoxical exasperation and at the same time orienting him or her toward a new, surprising perspective about the situation.

When the patients tried to cope with the complicated and elaborated rationalizations we had added, and with the absurd question as to the possibly positive meaning of their suffering, the results fell into two categories. In the second session, some patients reported something like this: "You know, doctor, I thought all week about what purpose my ideas and strange actions may have, but I haven't understood anything. However, I must say that my mind has been freer during the past few days." Others said, "Doctor, I think that I have understood that my actions really do serve some purpose, though I can't yet say what, but I must say that I have been a bit better and have had fewer fixations."

The effect of the paradoxical reframing was, therefore, to mitigate the obsessive tension — even if only a little — by complicating it even further, but also by implying an obscure, mysterious, and possibly positive aspect of the complaints. This permitted a shift of attention toward something different, so that instead of seeking not to think or act in a compulsive manner, the patient was able to concentrate on the possible usefulness of the symptoms, which, of course, was not defined. Paradoxically, the search for a positive explanation helped to mitigate the obsessive mechanism of "attempted solutions" — seeking not to think or do certain things, which only increased the obsessions. As we have said earlier, the willful effort to do something spontaneously inhibits spontaneity and renders that particular action impossible. The obsessive attempt to control obsessions produced the effect of maintaining and nourishing them. The reduction of even a small part of such a mechanism produced a rapid slackening of the tension.

In the second session, after the patient's report, we strengthened the hypothesis of a positive functional role of the symptoms by means of a series of outlandish ideas and suppositions. We followed this, toward the end of the session, with a paradoxical prescription, directed at the patient's compulsive behavior, formulated as follows: "All right, on the basis of what we have said so far, I am now going to assign you a specific task that you must carry out without asking questions or looking for explanations. This will help you to disperse any doubts about the positive role of your disorder, but you will have to get there yourself. I will give my explanations only afterward. Therefore, each time that you go to do the specific task that you are being asked to do, instead of resisting and not executing it, I want you to willingly repeat it ten times. Not one time more or less. Exactly ten times."

The prescription was given in the form of a hypnotic suggestion, in slow, repetitive, redundant language. The accountant who continually checked the growing number of invoices would have to check them ten times each time he felt the need to check; the young woman with nocturnal rituals would have to repeat them ten times; the young man obsessed by the fear of homosexuality would also have to look at all his magazines and at the most disturbing parts of the films ten times. Finally, the woman terrorized by the fear of having run over a pedestrian would have to return to the hypothetical scene of the crime ten times every time she experienced her doubt.

In the third session, the most frequent report was "Doctor, I carried out your assignment, but I did not succeed in doing it ten times. In fact, I was sometimes unable to do it at all. You told me that I would understand the function of my problems, but I still understand nothing." Several clients reported that they had not been capable of repeating the actions or rituals because they never felt the need to do them and could not force themselves to do what they were not willing to do; these patients also stated that they still did not understand the positive role of their problems.

The next therapeutic step was to emphasize the importance of carrying out the specific action exactly ten times; otherwise, the positive role of such symptoms could not be clarified and the clients would never gain control of them. Accordingly, the prescription was maintained for yet another week, underscoring the fact that the patient was beginning to assume control of the situation.

At the end of the third session, we told patients the following story as we accompanied them to the door: "There is an old story about an ant who asked a centipede — you know, those animals that move so well and elegantly with a hundred legs — 'Can you tell me how you can walk so smoothly with a hundred feet to move? Explain to me how you manage to control them all simultaneously.' The centipede began to think about it and then could no longer move or walk." After this brief story, the patients were invited to reflect on its significance and were sent on their way.

Second Stage: From the Fourth to the Sixth Session. In the fourth session, most patients reported feeling decisively better, having had fewer obsessions or compulsions that week, and they reported that each time they felt the impulse to engage in their symptomatic behavior, as soon as they started to execute it deliberately, the need to continue disappeared. In addition, many of these patients said that they had thought a lot about the centipede and had understood that they themselves had fallen into the same trap, but they did not realize why things were now changing. How was it possible that these uncontrollable impulses were diminishing or, in some cases, disappearing?

At this point we redefined the situation, explaining the trick that had been used and how the "be spontaneous" paradox may cause problems, but can also be used to resolve certain other problems — in this particular case, their own. In particular, we insisted on the obvious possibility of their using it to resolve such problems.

We also emphasized that it was now necessary to slow down the process of change: "If you step too heavily on the accelerator, you will go off the road." And also: "You know, I think that a relapse is likely within the next few weeks, because certain problems can return after having been resolved. So, be advised that in the coming days you will certainly have some sort of relapse; nevertheless, continue to do what I have recommended."

As we had expected, the following week only a few patients reported a relapse, the majority of them reporting that they not only had not experienced a relapse but actually felt a bit better, with fewer obsessions and almost no compulsive actions. The next move — after a redefinition of the situation and the obvious possibility of change and resolution of the problem — was to predict, in the case of those who had relapsed, another somewhat slighter relapse.

The following prescription was assigned to all: "Well, now that we have 'switched off' those troubling mechanisms, we can begin to use your sensibility and your attention in a positive way. For the next few days, when you go out, I want you to do what anthropologists do when they study a particular culture. They carefully observe modes of behavior — how individuals move, speak, act, and so forth — and on the basis of such observation they seek to understand such persons and the rules that govern their behavior, society, and culture. I want you to do just that, observing and studying the behavior of people whom you encounter. I want you to endeavor to understand, from their actions, what sorts of individuals they are. I am convinced that with your sensibility and powers of observation, you will discover some interesting things, which we will talk about in the next session."

This prescription, called the "prescription of the anthropologist," has as its objective the shifting of the patient's attention from self to others. That is to say, this maneuver helps patients avoid being too attentive to their own selves and actions. It is a mechanism that usually functions as a self-fulfilling prophecy, and shifts the patient's attention to the "anthropological" observation and study of others.

In the next session, the majority of patients reported no relapses and vividly described many different examples of human behavior. Indeed, the mass of information and reflections that the patients reported in their roles as "anthropologists" was surprising. Several related that they discerned behavioral symptoms in others and discovered that there were, in fact, many people with problems, something that they would not have believed before, thinking themselves the only ones to have them.

The session was spent entirely on reflections about patients' reports and the incentive to continue with this cognitive inquiry into the behavior of others, reinforcing the patients' ability to carry out this difficult task and emphasizing the tremendous utility of interacting with others.

Third Stage: From the Sixth Session Onward. In several cases, in the next session (normally the sixth or seventh), the obsessive problems were reduced to a minimum. Accordingly, we proceeded to a redefinition of the situation in order to emphasize the capability demonstrated by the patients in combatting their problems in collaboration with the therapist. In these cases, the time between sessions was lengthened, the intent being that of reinforcing the patients' autonomy. In successive sessions, we moved ahead with subsequent positive redefinitions of the situation and of the change obtained, until reaching the end of the therapy.

However, in the session after the second week of the "prescription of the anthropologist," the situation of most patients had undergone some change. They had reduced their obsessions to a minimum and were no longer enslaved to them, but they continued to think too much about specific things, complicating them, rendering them difficult and worrisome. Therefore, even if they were not exhibiting obsessive behavior, they maintained an obsessive inclination in their analysis of reality, thinking too much and acting too little.

We created a specific form of intervention for such situations: the prescription of the "magic formula."

In practice, tied to each of their ruminations was the obligation to write the following phrase in Engish five times: Think little and learn by doing!

The assignment was given with no discussion or explanation of the phrase's meaning. (Several patients knew English and understood the sentence immediately. The others were advised to have someone translate it for them.)

The prescription was to write the sentence "Think little and learn by doing" five times, on a sheet of paper given to them by the therapist, every time they found themselves thinking too much about a certain thing or situation.

No one carried out this prescription. It was because of this that the prescription was dubbed the "magic formula." Almost all of the patients related that, at the thought of having to write the sentence, they felt themselves liberated from thinking and rethinking things, and they began to act with more ease and less rumination.

It seems to us that this intervention is effective because of the irony it implies, and because the person who tries to execute such a task—after having made significant advances in fighting problems—will recognize it as a form of self-mockery. The patient will avoid this potential self-humiliation, and in avoiding it will also avoid the residual obsessiveness. At this point, even in these cases, we moved on to progressive positive redefinitions of the change achieved and of the capability the patient had demonstrated in confronting the problem. We began lengthening the interval between sessions until we reached the end of the therapy.

Fourth Stage: The Last Session. In the final session with obsessive patients, the same steps were taken as with phobic patients. We used detailed recapitulations, emphasizing the patient's personal capabilities as the key to change. Our main effort in the last meeting was to consolidate the patient's personal autonomy.

Efficacy and Effectiveness of the Treatment

The interventions described in this section were employed with twenty-four patients who suffered from obsessive disorders. The sample was composed of ten women and fourteen men, with a median age of twenty-nine, the youngest being seventeen years old and the oldest being fifty-one. The social standings of the patients were varied, as were their occupations: they were clerks, teachers, professionals, doctors, business people, students, and so on. One particularity of this sample was that it included no housewives. Although the sample included a wide array of personalities with a common symptomatology, the number of cases it comprises is insufficient to yield statistically significant conclusions.

Efficacy. We used the same parameters in evaluation of the efficacy of treatments for obsessive disorders as we used with the treatments for phobic disorders. The results, displayed in Table 5.3, were as follows:

> Seventeen cases were completely resolved: there was complete resolution of the problem at the end of the therapy and absence of relapse within the space of a year.
>
> No case was considerably improved: in no case was remission of symptoms complete at the end of therapy, with sporadic but slight relapses reported at the follow-up.
>
> Six cases showed little improvement: there was partial reduction of the symptomatology at the end of treatment, with subsequent rather frequent moments of obsessiveness, which nevertheless were described by the patients as considerably less intense or frequent than prior to treatment.
>
> One case was unchanged: therapy was interrupted after ten sessions because it had not produced any change whatsoever.
>
> No case worsened: following treatment, no case showed a worsening of the problem reported at the beginning of therapy.

Table 5.3. Efficacy of Treatment of Obsessive Disorders.

Case	Cases	
Outcome	N	%
Resolved	17	71
Much improved	-	-
Little improved	6	25
Unchanged	1	4
Worsened	-	-
Total	24	100

Effectiveness. The median duration of the therapy was 16.1 sessions, from a minimum of 7 sessions for the briefest treatment, to a maximum of 31 sessions for the longest. In order to offer a clearer picture of the effectiveness of therapy, we have subdivided the cases that were resolved or considerably improved into three subgroups: therapy lasting from 7 to 10 sessions, from 11 to 20 sessions, and from 21 to 30 sessions (see Table 5.4).

From this breakdown of the data we see that about 94 percent of the cases were treated in fewer than 20 sessions.

Table 5.4. Median Duration of Treatment for Obsessive Disorders.

Total Number	Cases Resolved or Much Improved	
of Sessions	N	%
7–10	9	53
11–20	7	41
21–30	1	6

Note: Median duration of treatment = 16.1 sessions.

Reflections on the Results

The data relative to the results obtained by the application of our therapeutic model to obsessive disorders shows a satisfactory efficacy. In 71 percent of the cases, patients achieved complete remission of their symptoms by the end of therapy, and these patients had no relapses. Noteworthy, in comparison to the treatment of phobic disorders, are the little-improved cases and the one entirely unchanged case.

With regard to effectiveness (the time employed to obtain results), this treatment method has decisively positive results, particularly in comparison with the usual psychotherapeutic timeframe for the disorders in question. In fact, 94 percent of the cases with a positive result were treated in fewer than twenty sessions.

To conclude this chapter, it seems important to reflect on the epistemological relevance in psychotherapy. Any discipline that wishes to assert the scientific rigor of its research methodology must put its techniques for study and intervention into practice and use them to achieve practical objectives. It most certainly must not adapt objectives to its theories and techniques. From this perspective, the conviction so often held by psychotherapists that the same rigid psychotherapeutic techniques can be applied to every type of mental and behavioral problem strikes us as absurd. We believe that only specific treatment approaches fitted to specific disorders can be fruitfully utilized, and not universal panaceas. Finally, we also believe that future psychotherapeutic research must address the study and practice of ever more efficacious and efficient specific programs of treatment.

Chapter 6

Four Case Examples

In this chapter, we describe some specific interventions devised for patients who presented unique problems. Apart from the strategies and techniques presented in the previous chapter, the possibilities for devising useful interventions are open to thoughtful and resourceful therapists. At times, a patient's special needs and particular context will call for something out of the ordinary. Unusual techniques can spark the creative flash that upsets the patient's rigid pathological system, opening it to change.

Original interventions often give rise to innovative strategic therapies that are applicable — with appropriate adaptation — to diverse problem situations. This kind of development is at the heart of a scientific discipline, in which the context of justification is as indispensable as the context of discovery.

First Case: Therapy Outside the Usual Setting

Our first clinical case involves a somewhat unusual therapeutic intervention that will undoubtedly provoke reactions from readers who are firmly convinced of the absolute necessity of a regular setting for psychotherapy.

I was invited to a city in northern Italy to give a series of lectures to teachers. At the end of one of these lectures, one of the teachers requested a private interview. She was a young woman of twenty-two, and for about two years had been suffering from frequent panic attacks, which totally incapacitated her, and occasional fainting spells. She said that these problems began after a series of very frightening medical examinations, to

which she had had to submit because of a suspected grave illness (which had been medically ruled out). Ever since, she had
begun to have outbursts of panic. These were becoming stronger
and more frequent, to the point where several months ago she
had had to stop working. Our first response to this woman was
that it would be difficult to intervene because of the distance
between our cities. But the woman was not discouraged and
insisted that she would go to any length for treatment. We offered
to refer her to colleagues closer to her home, but she was so
insistent that, almost as a joke, we decided to try something unusual. We said, "Perhaps we can resolve your problems quickly
and without too much traveling on your part. For our lectures,
we will have to come here six more times. Before or after the
lectures we can meet, perhaps have a bite to eat, and conduct
your therapy."

The woman was astonished, but agreed to this unusual
suggestion. And so, in the lecture hall's antechamber, her treatment began.

In the manner of the procedure for treating phobias presented in the last chapter, the first reframing of the problem
was done (instilling fear of help), and the first behavioral prescription, the keeping of a log, was given. The second meeting
took place two weeks later, in a restaurant over dinner. The
woman mentioned having written in the log several times con-
comitantly with the panic attacks, although the attacks had been
less frequent than usual. She then said that she became aware
that in writing about these episodes, her anxiety and fear were
reduced. Finally, she indicated that she was refraining from asking her family and fiancé for help. We went on to redefine the
situation in the usual way by emphasizing that the problems
no longer appeared as invincible or inescapable as they had at
first. Finally, we gave the following prescriptions: (1) continue
to keep the log, (2) practice self-induced anxiety every day for
half an hour. (See the section in Chapter Five on the second
stage of treatment for phobic disorders.)

The third meeting took place in the lecture hall's antechamber, about ten days later. The patient related that she had
had only two panic attacks since our last meeting, both of which

were minor, and both of which she had controlled by writing about them in her log. Concerning the half-hour anxiety prescription, she said that after trying to force herself to think of her anxiety and of the fear of feeling it for a short time, her mind took an entirely different direction. She had found herself thinking of enjoyable things and happy times of her life.

We then proceeded with the usual redefinition of the problem and of the effects provoked by the prescriptions. We discussed the strengthening of her faith in the concrete, demonstrated possibility of resolving her symptoms. The two behavioral prescriptions were maintained (as described in Chapter Five, second and third stages).

Two weeks later, we met again. The woman related that since our last encounter she had not suffered any panic episodes; she had had some isolated moments of anxiety, but she had not bothered to record them because they seemed so slight in comparison to her preceding difficulties. She also related that during the daily half-hour anxiety exercise she was still unsuccessful in conjuring up her fears; rather, all the positive things that she wanted to do came to mind.

At this point, after having redefined the situation as decisively changed in view of her demonstrated ability, we proceeded to eliminate the two prescriptions. We suggested that she take up her scholastic work again, and assigned her the task of carrying out the "prescription of the anthropologist" (described in Chapter Five) both at school, with her colleagues and students, and with her relatives, friends, and any strangers she might meet.

Our final session took place about two weeks later, again at a restaurant over a meal. The woman related that she had gone back to work without any difficulty. She found that attending to her students — observing and studying them — had stimulated in her a number of positive reflections, and that in observing and studying her colleagues she had discovered several strange aspects to some of them, which helped her to appreciate that she need not feel herself the sole "rare beast."

At this point, the situation's radical change was redefined, and the usual strategy of the final session was applied (see Chapter

Five, fourth stage). We asked only that the woman telephone after one month to report on her situation. She called, punctually, saying that she had suffered no panic attacks and felt as well as she ever had in her life.

It is clear that no reliable conclusion can be drawn from a single case. But we believe that this example is cause for reflection on the fact that, to obtain change, the traditional setting of psychotherapy — with its rigid schedule, the office with chaise or couch, the suffused light, and so on — is not indispensable. Freud himself demonstrated this point in the solution of Mahler's psychosexual problems. In fact, Freud cured Mahler's problems — they were great friends — in one whole day spent together, dining together and strolling through Vienna (Fachinelli, 1983). In this case, Freud broke his own norms relative to the psychoanalytic setting, effecting a splendid — brief and specific — therapeutic intervention.

Second Case: Reframing the Meaning of Brotherhood

When a psychiatrist in his fifties applied to our center to undergo training, a critical situation emerged during the first conversations, and his request for training became a request for help. The situation was as follows. The man was unable to get married; his morbid submission, first to a castrating mother and then to an older unmarried sister (who, after the death of their mother, had assumed the role of the family authority), had prevented him from taking this step. In fact, after the death of the sister, he practiced the same morbid submission with regard to his younger brother, who suffered from paranoid disturbances.

The two brothers had been raised to be unquestioningly submissive to their mother and sister. Subsequently, every woman they expressed interest in collided with this family background because they could not stand either the sister's aggressiveness or, sooner or later, the mother's controlling and overbearing attitude. The brothers were thus unable to lead effective lives of their own. In addition, the psychiatrist revealed that his brother was a paranoiac, who displayed delusions of euphoria and omnipotence, and whose hyperactivity occasionally gave way to deep depression.

Two years after the death of their sister, the paranoid brother assumed her role as the dominant family figure. He intervened in a violent and explosive way each time his brother tried to establish an affective relationship. He justified his interventions into his brother's private life by claiming that the women his brother found were not worthy of him. He described them as being insubstantial, superficial, and interested only in money and the brother's social position. He believed he had to intervene on his brother's behalf, to keep him from harming himself.

In the last few years, the psychiatrist had been involved in a tormented relationship with a woman who had initially suffered the older sister's outrages, and now those of the younger brother. Each encounter between them was disastrous. The situation escalated to the point of our patient's having to choose between remaining with his morbid family system and abandoning his companion, or breaking with that system and throwing himself into the other relationship. The situation was complicated when the two brothers were left alone after the death of the sister because the psychiatrist was well aware of his brother's problems and feared for his mental collapse in the event of a break between them. In other words, he felt himself crushed by the emotional blackmail under which his brother unwittingly held him. The psychiatrist, however, firmly held on to his affective relationship with the woman, which — considering his advanced age — he believed would be his last chance to build a family. For her part, the woman pressed the fact that he would have to choose whether to be with her definitively and under the same roof, or end their relationship and stay with his "little brother."

Our psychiatrist found himself in the proverbial situation of the donkey standing in the middle of a river with its saddlebags full of sponges that are growing heavier as they absorb more and more water. The donkey cannot decide whether to go on to the bank ahead or turn back, and ends up being swept away by the current. In the face of such a dilemma, the first therapeutic maneuver was to explore the nature of the morbid relationship

between the two brothers so as to understand what kinds of
strategies might produce change.

The psychiatrist was treating his brother — who was una-
ware of his mental illness — in a modest and nonauthoritative
way with medications, putting up with his mania and his hyperactivity, and preferring not to reveal to the brother his diagnosis. The brother, however, in his impetuous euphoria and delusions of omnipotence, completely dominated their social lives,
leading a professional life of utter chaos amid problems that were
deftly and silently smoothed over by the psychiatrist brother.
Practically speaking, the situation appeared truly paradoxical
in that the paranoid brother was the one who possessed the real
power to manage their life together and to meddle, without hesi-
tation, in both the private life and the professional career of the
psychiatrist brother. It was the paranoid younger brother who
pushed the older one to take classes and to participate in sym-
posia, and who intended to find an appropriate companion for
him. And it was the younger brother who, in his delirium of
omnipotence, destructively assumed control of whatever social
activity either of them happened to pursue.

The therapy developed in the following manner: It was
agreed with the psychiatrist that we would attempt a maneuver
for which both brothers would have to be present at the next
session. He would tell his brother that this meeting was necessary for his (the psychiatrist's) training, without revealing the
therapeutic scope of the meeting. What follows is a transcript
of several of the most salient parts of the session (which was
videotaped), synthesized with material from successive meetings.

The conversation began with the therapist explaining to
the younger brother the elder's motive for convening the meeting, saying that it was indispensable for his therapeutic training. He continued by explaining that the psychiatrist's problems of insecurity and emotional instability prevented him from
successfully exercising his profession and required, for their resolution, the younger brother's assistance.

The brother was initally surprised by these statements and
criticized himself for his exuberance ("When I state my opinion
it overwhelms him. I just take off, and he — who is an introvert —

succumbs"). But then he insisted that this attitude toward his brother was necessary. He spoke of his brother's love life, saying that he had "wasted" eight years with a nurse who lacked both character and culture, and that was why he — the younger brother — felt the need to find a more fitting companion for his brother. The therapist interrupted him and asked him questions about his private life. The younger brother spoke of having spent several years with a married woman, and the therapist asked him if they were "wasted" years. When he answered no, he was asked why they had such different views of their respective private lives. The next step was the reframing of the different characters of the two brothers.

Therapist: *(Turning to the dominant brother)* From our talk, it seems clear to me that you and your brother function in two entirely different ways and have two very different styles of communication. You are very strong, exuberant, affirmative; your brother is introverted, yielding, and accommodating. It is obvious that your brother feels overwhelmed by you.

The difference between you is similar to that between a cruise ship and a freight barge. The cruiser is powerful and fast, and the freight barge is a slow boat, capable of carrying great loads but not moving at high speeds.

Imagine yourself as a cruise ship towing a freight barge. If the cruiser accelerates too quickly, the barge cannot adjust to the speed. It could break apart or spill its load, or sink. *(Pause)* For example, you have taken up the subject of women. Steady, don't go so fast! *(Pause)* Calm and understanding are necessary because if not . . .

Younger brother: We damage each other in turn.

Therapist: You damage each other.

Younger brother: For example, the woman that I am looking for . . .

Therapist: Fine! But it is clear that your brother must like that woman.

Younger brother: Of course, he will want her. The problem is that he is now with someone else, and I am not sure how to make him break up with that worthless woman.

Therapist: You could do it. But if your brother is currently experiencing something that he finds valuable, why would you want to deprive him of that? You spent years with the wrong woman. And yet you got something out of that experience, didn't you?

Younger brother: I think so, yes!

Therapist: Now your brother is in a similar situation. And you are now like the cruiser towing the barge: if you go too fast, you could overwhelm and wreck it.

Younger brother: Well, then, we must not speak . . .

Therapist: No, only with a different, more flexible attitude. Fortunately, we are all different from each other; we need to learn to respect this diversity, its rhythms. At times it is difficult to accept that others are different from us, particularly when we are close to them.

Younger brother: I would like to see my brother with a woman who could fill —

Therapist: Excuse me, but are you currently involved with a woman?

Younger brother: No.

Therapist: Doesn't your brother think that you feel lonely? He at least has a woman in his life.

Younger brother: Yes . . . I think of it . . .

Therapist: You need to create a more open family. Your life together has created ties that are too strong, even though they are also beautiful. But to be able to continue like this, or rather in growing . . .

Younger brother: Great respect is needed.

Therapist: Reciprocal availability. Do you understand?

Younger brother: Yes.

Therapist: And don't insist too much on the woman problem. "Reciprocal availability" also means not always speaking yourself, but allowing your brother to have his say. *(Pause)* The first time that you both came to therapy, your brother didn't say a word.

Younger brother: True.

Therapist: Keep the cruiser and the barge in mind: people go to help only if they are asked and are not overwhelmed.

Younger brother: Then I wouldn't have had to come. If I hadn't urged him, he would never have come. I understand. My task is to encourage but never to overpower him. That is the key.

Therapist: Exactly. Stimulate, but never overpower. I suggest this because of your brother's insecurity and instability. Otherwise, he cannot become an effective therapist.

Younger brother: How much time will it take for him to confront these problems?

Therapist: Don't expect immediate magical solutions. I spoke of slow steps. Think it over. *(Pause)* You must also look for solutions yourself. *(Pause)* We must, together, find the right way. I ask for your collaboration, because I believe that it will serve you both well.

At the following session, the psychiatrist enthusiastically related that during the intervening week his brother had not interfered with his affective life and had not been depressed or aggressive, but had been particularly helpful and attentive.

At this point I told the psychiatrist to go on a vacation with his companion so as to verify the reactions of his brother, with whom the following intervention was carried out at the next session:

Therapist: Very good! You have proven yourself to be capable of handling the situation. I've begun to see a greater assertiveness in your brother, for which he should be grateful to you insofar as you have helped him to reassume responsibility for himself.

Younger brother: Thanks, doctor. You have made me think, and I am happy that my brother has become more courageous. But with this woman . . .

Therapist: Yes, I wanted to speak with you about her. I believe that you should try to find a better woman for your brother, but until you have found her, let him play a bit more with his present darling. All right?

Younger brother: Agreed. You'll see, I will find him the right woman.

After the vacation, the psychiatrist returned, saying that his brother had behaved very well. He had not "intentionally" fallen ill in his absence, as he had always done when he had felt "abandoned." This tactic had forced the elder brother to come home immediately from previous trips. But this time, they had remained in touch with frequent but pleasant telephone calls.

At this point I suggested to the psychiatrist that he organize, if possible, a dinner with his brother, his companion, and a woman friend of hers. The psychiatrist was fearful that such a proposal would lead to his brother's refusal to attend or, worse, to an explosion at the dinner table between his brother and his companion. However, we pressed the importance of arranging such an evening.

At the next session, the psychiatrist reported that the dinner had taken place and that the evening had taken an extraordinary turn. His brother had quickly warmed to his companion's friend, was quite kind to her, and throughout the evening maintained a convivial atmosphere with wit and sparkling vitality. Not only that, the group had met again during the course of the week, and the younger brother had suggested to the psychiatrist that they invite the women to their home for a more intimate evening soon.

At this point, the final touch to this particular therapeutic intervention was to see the domineering brother again. We complimented him on his collaboration in the solution of his psychiatrist brother's problems, who — having achieved greater emotional stability and assertiveness — would be able to pursue the training he had initially requested.

No reference was made to the women, to the dinner parties, or to the total reversal of the initial situation (after all, it was the older brother who had "found the right woman" for the younger one). The psychiatrist now had the possibility of pursuing his own private life without abandoning his brother. Indeed, the brothers had found a new form of complicity: masculine complicity in the courtship game. With this new relational foundation, their situation was radically changed.

We believe that this intervention in a specific human problem exemplifies the following points: (a) one can intervene in problems without explaining the action one hopes to accomplish, (b) there is unexpected power in the art of reframing and in small, indirect interventions, and (c) it is necessary, at times fundamental, to prescribe limited goals. In fact, in this case we were not at all anxious to work directly and in a specific way on the paranoia of the younger brother, or to search for a deep and definitive cure. We concentrated instead on making a concrete change in the relationship pattern between the two brothers — on helping them relate to each other in a happier way. Thus, the intervention was limited to the change of an unproductive interpersonal situation.

Third Case: On the Usefulness of Error

The third case deals with the application of a particular kind of prescription frequently utilized in the treatment of obsessive patients. The interesting thing about this intervention is that it was the result of a diagnostic error; in fact, the treatment was based on this wrong diagnosis. No therapy is infallible (although many therapists do not like to admit this), and we believe that to accept and analyze one's own mistakes leads to a broadening of one's capacity for intervention. In this case, the error led us to reject some classical treatment modalities, and this led to the bizarre, creative flash that produced the solution of the problem. Without the initial mistake, we would not have been forced to innovate. On the basis of this experience, we believe that error, if accepted by the therapist, can at times be a means to discovery and a push toward a solution.

The case is that of a twenty-six-year-old woman coming to us because she had not been able to work for almost two weeks. Strong fits of anxiety and immobilizing panic attacks had made it impossible for her to pursue her work as a bookkeeper. She described her difficulties with a surprising command of clinical language and concepts, describing a perfect phobic symptomatology and giving detailed and exhaustive examples of her panic attacks and her fits of anxiety. She mentioned that she had studied her symptoms in several psychology books.

The therapist was taken in by this seemingly perfect self-diagnosis and immediately began to apply the appropriate therapeutic actions, following the procedure for the treatment of phobic disorders described in Chapter Five.

At the second session the woman reported that she felt a bit better and that recording her panic attacks in the log had assuaged them. She gave the therapist her written record of the first session, full of notes, together with another list that she had made entirely on her own. Though this surprised us, we gave it little weight and proceeded with the usual treatment of phobic disorders.

At the third session, the patient related that her symptoms continued to lessen in both frequency and intensity but brought, just the same, two filled notebooks. The therapist told the woman that she should discontinue keeping the diary and went ahead with the usual therapy, which included prescribing a half-hour daily session of self-induced anxiety (see Chapter Five).

At the fourth session, the patient reported having been unable to force herself to feel ill or anxious, notwithstanding her efforts to think of the worst situations or fantasies; rather, she said she found them ridiculous. In addition, she revealed that she was feeling ready to try to go back to work. The odd thing was that, although this prescription had been canceled two sessions before, she again brought to this session two diaries completely filled with notes. She said that writing them made her feel decisively better; they allowed her to unburden herself.

At this point the therapist had some doubts, partly because in reading the diaries he realized that she had noted not only critical episodes but everything that passed through her mind: all her thoughts, emotions, and ideas. Nevertheless, since the symptomatic situation was improving, the therapist continued to follow the usual treatment.

At the fifth session, the patient related that she had gone back to work without any great problems; she had suffered some short episodes of anxiety, but had controlled them. She once again produced her diaries, full of notes. In response to the therapist's question about the function of such a tiring daily exercise, she said, "You know, doctor, it is very important for me to write, even if it is tiresome and time-consuming, because I have found that in writing I can control my fears. I feel that writing keeps my frightful ideas at a distance, as if in writing I can keep certain things away."

At this point the therapist had an insight regarding the woman's behavior, which seemed incongruent with the diagnosis of phobia and with the usual reactions of such a patient to treatment: he realized that he was dealing with an obsessive patient. She had not ceased writing her diaries because she was convinced that if she did, her fears and panic attacks would return. In other words, the writing of the diaries had been transformed into an obsessive ritual to keep her symptoms away. This realization opened the way to a better understanding of several aspects of the woman's personal life that had been neglected earlier owing to the treatment's (as reported by the woman) having been so successful. In fact, it turned out that the woman's phobic crises had resulted from her having felt compelled to perform several repetitive behavior rituals every day for the past several years. These made her extremely insecure, forcing her to check everything many times. Eventually, they prevented her from ever feeling certain or calm about anything regarding her own actions, and it was at that point that the panic attacks began.

The panic attacks were merely the most explosive symptom

of the obsessive root of the woman's problems. The initial diagnostic hypothesis — misguided by the patient's self-diagnosis — was not appropriate. The treatment based on this diagnosis had led to concrete improvements in the woman's behavior through the prescription of an "obsessive ritualization." This, however, could not be considered a success; if the ritual were removed, the situation would almost certainly collapse again. At this point, the therapist was confused, not knowing how to untangle a situation whose intricacies he had complicated through his own intervention. He decided to take his time, without mentioning to the woman what he had realized, saying to her only that if she found it useful, she should continue to write and to bring in the logs.

The problem in this situation was how to deal with the obsession without upsetting the small behavioral adjustment obtained through the treatment; how to eliminate the obsessive ritual, produced by the therapy, without creating new problems? In the midst of these tortuous reflections, an idea — as bizarre as it was to be efficacious — came to the therapist's mind.

At the next session, after listening to the woman's self-report (she was pleased with her progressively improving situation), and after having received the two latest logs, overflowing with notes, the therapist said, "Very well, but we can do even more. To this end, you must, as usual, follow to the letter the task that I am going to give you. Considering how important writing down your thoughts and ideas and describing your emotions and crises has been for you, I assign you the task of writing ten times — in the notebook I'll now give you — whenever the urge to write something for me comes on, the sentence that I will now write on the first page of the notebook. For now, as usual, don't ask me any questions; I will explain the assignment after you have completed it." Then the therapist wrote on the first page of the notebook "Think little and learn by doing!"

At the seventh session, the woman returned annoyed and said that she felt she was being treated "like an idiot." In writing the sentence and considering its meaning she realized its stupidity. Consequently, she had carried out the assignment only twice and then destroyed those pages. Since then, whenever she wanted to write something for the therapist, she automatically felt herself an idiot and could not write anything. The prescription — notwithstanding the indignant reaction of the patient — was maintained for another week without explanation.

At the eighth session, the patient reported not having written anything at all and not having had even the desire to write. But the most important thing was that over the intervening two weeks the patient had continued to boost her well-being; she said that she felt fine and had experienced only sporadic anxiety attacks, which she had easily controlled. This had been accomplished without the obsessive ritual of writing entries in the log book.

The therapy went on for two additional sessions (at longer intervals), which dealt mostly with the final redefinition of the personal autonomy acquired by the patient.

We can conclude the presentation of this case by emphasizing the necessity of continually evaluating any therapeutic intervention. If the intervention is not successful, one must have the mental flexibility and capacity to modify and reorient it according to the nature of the case. As in the case just described, this can lead to the application of new, successful strategies. Error, like disorder, becomes a disjunctive element that can — if accepted and utilized — establish new, more efficacious balances within a system — in this case, a therapeutic system.

Fourth Case: "Advertising" Instead of Concealing

A man of twenty-nine — tall, blond, handsome, interesting, wealthy, and successful with women — presented himself with a request for help with a problem he described as "dramatic." He said that for about a year he had been unable to have a satisfactory erection, and so had not been able to engage in sexual relationships. The man could not explain how this problem might have started, considering that he had had numerous lovers and fully satisfying sexual relationships in the past. Lately, however, whenever he was about to perform the sex act, he would have a normal erection until the moment of penetration, when his penis would go limp, leaving him dismayed, embarrassed, and humiliated.

Our "playboy" also related that he had been in treatment for some time with a sexologist, who had prescribed various techniques, such as prolonged abstention before a sexual encounter, penetration in spite of insufficient erection, manual and oral stimulation by the partner, intercourse in the strangest positions, and the use of aphrodisiacs. None of this had produced any result; whenever he attempted penetration, he lost his erection. He was in a state of deep depression and obsession regarding his problem and was convinced of the impossibility of resolving it, considering all the failed efforts attempted until then.

Discussion during the initial session revealed that the problem had begun when the patient had read in a newspaper article that all so-called playboys (men who have many sexual relationships without necessarily being in love—living as if playing a superficial game) would eventually become either impotent or premature ejaculators. According to the theory expounded in the article, such persons would sooner or later develop psychosexual problems. From that moment, he began to worry about such a possibility and to have doubts about his sexual performance. As the reader might well understand, he began to ruminate about his performance each time that he had sex, finally finding himself suffering the classical effect of the "be spontaneous" paradox. In other words—as in the story of the centipede that cannot walk when it tries consciously to move each of its hundred feet—the patient, upon monitoring his spontaneous sexual responses closely, wound up inhibiting them. And so he entered into the paradoxical game of always checking his performance more closely and therefore inhibiting himself more deeply, eventually arriving at the point where his worries became facts. In other words, the prophecy had fulfilled itself. (For a description of the mechanism of self-fulfilling prophecies, see Watzlawick, 1984, pp. 95–116.)

This diagnostic hypothesis was confirmed by the fact that in the preliminary phases of lovemaking all would go well, and his erection would be quite strong until he attempted penetration (which for him was the real proof of erectile capacity). Then he would lose the erection, and all his practical or imaginative efforts to regain it were useless.

At this point, the problem was understood and the young man's attempted solutions, which exacerbated it, had been identified. The specific behavioral circumstances of the problem situation became the next subject of exploration. Recently, he had avoided any sexual encounter whatsoever for fear of being humiliated again by his failure. If he found himself alone with a woman he invented excuses and fled the situation, driven by fear and becoming increasingly depressed by these experiences. In addition, a grotesque aspect of his predicament was that, since he was handsome and desirable, his avoidance of sexual intimacy was seen by the women concerned as intriguing behavior, thus strikingly increasing their interest in him. Thus he found himself in a paradoxical situation: women were drawn to him by his mysterious unavailability, while he continued to flee from them, fearful of having to reveal his impotence.

The following intervention was made in the course of the third session:

Therapist: Very well, I believe that I now understand your problem and that we can do something about resolving it, but I don't know if you will be in a position to do what I would like to ask of you. Nevertheless, I am going to suggest something that could help you, provided that you follow to the letter what I recommend.

Patient: I would do anything to resolve my problem, doctor, tell me and I will do it!

Therapist: Fine. I want you to do the following until we meet again in two weeks: You must go out with three different women within the space of these two weeks. For you it won't be difficult to find three women, I would imagine. You must take each of them out to an elegant and intimate place, for a delicious candlelight supper. You will create a romantic and seductive atmosphere, about which I have little to teach you, considering your vast experience! After dinner, later in the evening, you must press on to initiate a sexual relationship, but — and this is crucial — after a bit of preliminary lovemaking, you must stop and completely reveal your problem in detail, apologizing to your partner for the fact that you will surely not succeed in providing her a satisfying erotic experience. Then, considering the fact that by now your partner is aware of your trouble and you have no further reason to worry about a poor performance, go ahead and try to have sex. You will already have revealed your problem and you won't have any reason to be ashamed; you might find at least a little pleasure if you try.

Patient: But, doctor, you are asking me to reveal my impotence. Then everyone will know.

Therapist: Well, I said that I wasn't sure that you were prepared to do what I was asking of you, and perhaps you really are not.

Patient: No, I didn't mean that. If it will help, I'll do it. Sooner or later, everyone would know anyway.

As the reader will have already understood, to the patient's paradoxical situation an even more paradoxical prescription was applied. The obligation to reveal his impotence meant unveiling the terrible and embarrassing secret, but it also relieved the tension of having to succeed at all costs, and of imposing on himself the paradox of trying to be intentionally spontaneous in achieving an erection — an effort that usually has an inhibiting effect. Revealing the problem, however, counteracts the "attempted solutions," and produces emotional relaxation and the free expression of the spontaneous behavioral response — in this case, the erection.

This is exactly how it worked out for the patient, who at the fourth session was almost incredulous at having been capable of highly satisfactory and prolonged intercourse with all three women. He was astonished by the fact that, after having revealed his shameful problem of impotence, he was capable of marvelous and, contrary to what he had revealed, sustained potency. The women felt as if he had fooled them with stories of impotence, and were convinced that this must have been one of his seductive tricks to excite them even more. He said that all three women were quite struck by his confession and showed great sweetness and openness, which made the erotic situations even more tender and beautiful.

We then explained the intervention to the patient. After this session, there were two follow-ups, the first after two weeks and the next a month later, at which time the therapy was terminated.

We believe that this case is an example of how at times very simple maneuvers or strategies can produce very great effects, provided that they put pressure on the patterns of behavior that maintain the problem.

We not did inquire into what morbid relation the young man might have had with his mother, or what terrible childhood traumas he might have suffered, or what doubts our patient had about his sexual identity. Rather, we were interested in finding the solution to his specific problem. If, after solving the immediate problem, the patient desires to undertake the long interior search for the numerous possible and hypothetical "whys," or causal explanations, there will always be time to do so, but only after being liberated from the problem itself.

Chapter 7

Outcome Research

Learning to bear clearly in mind that no one is perfectly happy is perhaps the most direct way to achieve happiness. Of course, no one is perfectly happy, but there are many levels to our suffering; this is illness.

—G. C. Lichtenberg, *The Little Book of Consolation*

One of the most frequent criticisms of the strategic approach is the lack of data relative to its results. Researchers involved in the comparative evaluation of the results of various kinds of therapy complain that strategic therapists have never systematically presented their findings. Such criticism suggests that the strategic approach seems too miraculous or magical to be considered a repeatable and reliable therapeutic model. Strategic therapists have been rightly accused of paying little attention and giving scarce importance to the conventional presentation of their data along the usual lines of psychological and social research. And it is true that the strategists have preferred to give ample space to innovative theoretical perspectives and to the description of sometimes eccentric kinds of therapeutic interventions, which in comparison with other therapeutic procedures can often seem too effective, and almost magical.

What might even further astonish an outside observer is the way in which the systemic approach and its strategic evolution—based on a rigorous methodology of observation (the use of videorecording, the one-way mirror, observers)—may seem to be inadequate regarding the evaluation and systematic presentation of its results. It could certainly be said that strategic therapy has snubbed the research community's requirements for the presentation of its findings. Few and far between

116

are efforts at systematically presenting the results of strategic therapy, as Weakland, Fisch, and Watzlawick did in 1974.

The disparity between the quantity of literature about the theory and practice of systemic and strategic therapy and the lack of published systematic results is mirrored by the absence of direct reference to it in the literature of comparative outcome studies. The few data describing strategic therapy either are not taken into account because of their scarcity or are incorporated into the data relative to the results of other therapies. (For the most recent comparative research on therapeutic results, see Garfield, 1980, and Sirigatti, 1988.)

Sirigatti has suggested that if the systemic and strategic therapists want their results to be taken seriously by researchers, they must present them to the scientific community according to the methodology of social research, in such a way that they are also comparable to the data for other kinds of therapy (personal communication, Siena, 1988). Recognizing the legitimacy of these objections, in the following pages we will present an evaluation of the results of strategic therapy conducted with a large and heterogeneous group of patients.

Methodological Criteria

Before moving on to the presentation and discussion of the data, it is important first to present the methodological criteria of this inquiry, which will illuminate the epistemological choices underlying those criteria.

The Concept of Efficacy

The evaluation of the effects or results obtained in therapy is, without a doubt, one of the thorniest issues in psychotherapy. Much of the difficulty arises from the different schools of psychotherapy having different criteria for establishing the efficacy of therapy, with the unavoidable consequence of diverse theoretical perspectives, which at times assume opposing positions. For example, a Jungian analyst will see the efficacy of therapy in the achievement of personal "individuation," while for a behaviorist it will be the "extinction" of behavioral symptoms.

These are only two of numerous examples of the conceptual disparity in the objectives of therapy and in the evaluation of the efficacy or inefficacy of treatment. It is understandable that different theories of the human personality also provide for different objectives, and that such differences result in different evaluation methods. Once again, our perceptions and conceptions determine our observations.

In other words, it is the specific theoretical formulation of "human nature" that determines the definition of sane or insane, normal or pathological, and — consequently — the notion of "recovery" and the goals of therapy. There are many different formulations of "recovery" and of the efficacy of treatment, but, as Sirigatti notes (1988, p. 230), there seems to be some agreement in defining a specific treatment as effective when it leads to any of the following:

> Symptom improvement
> Increased ability to work
> Better sexual adjustment
> Improvement in interpersonal relations
> Increased ability to confront common psychological difficulties
> Increased ability to react to daily stress

The strategic approach, as illustrated in Chapter Two, is not concerned with a theory that can succinctly describe the concepts of normality and abnormality, nor with an all-embracing theory of "human nature." Rather, it is tied to the constructivist philosophy of knowledge, which — based on the idea of the irreducibility of human nature and behavior to a single, comprehensive description and explanation — is concerned with the appropriate means of making the individual's relationship with "reality" more functional. From such a theoretical perspective, the efficacy of therapy is represented by the resolution of the patient's specific problem.

The concept of "recovery" does not entail a complete absence of problems, but rather the overcoming of a specific problem experienced by the patient in a specific timeframe and context of his or her life. Therefore, the evaluation of the effects of strategic therapy can certainly be considered to be in agreement with the criteria listed above, with the caveat that no absolute generalization can be defined, and that success or the lack of it will be ascertained in relation to the initial therapeutic objectives. Accordingly, success will involve the solution of the patient's presenting problem and the achievement of goals that were agreed upon at the outset of therapy.

Success or lack of success can have many dimensions; therefore, it is important to consider not only the categories of "resolved" or "unresolved" cases, but also the categories relative to cases that are "considerably improved" or "little improved," and it is also crucial to evaluate the possibility of deterioration following the end of therapy (see Sirigatti, 1988, p. 221). The criteria for establishing efficacy used in this evaluative inquiry are defined below.

The Concept of Effectiveness

To evaluate the efficacy of the treatment, we used two sets of parameters. One is the effectiveness of the treatment (the evaluation of the outcome of therapy). Were the goals that patient and therapist agreed upon at the beginning of therapy achieved? Were the patient's problems resolved at the end of therapy? Was there a shift in the original symptom? The second is the efficacy of treatment over time. Were the results of therapy maintained over time, or was there a relapse? Have new problems replaced the original ones?

Three follow-up sessions were arranged for three months, six months, and one year after the end of treatment. The follow-up sessions were conducted as interviews with the patient and his family or partner; the interviews were conducted along the lines established by Sirigatti (1988).

We consider a case resolved and the treatment completely successful only when, in addition to fulfilling the first set of parameters, the second set of parameters is also fulfilled — that is, when the disappearance of symptoms and problems at the end of therapy is maintained over time, without relapses or substitution of new symptoms for the original ones.

The evaluation of the effects of therapy is based on five categories of results:

> Resolved cases: complete resolution of the problem at the end of therapy and absence of relapses within one year.
>
> Considerably improved cases: complete remission of symptoms at the end of therapy, but with subsequent sporadic and slight relapses.
>
> Little-improved cases: partial remission of symptoms at the end of therapy, with occasional crises and recurrence of the symptoms reported at follow-up. However, such problems were generally described as being considerably less serious than those before therapy.
>
> Unchanged cases: treatment accomplished no significant change in the patient's situation after ten sessions. In these cases, treatment ended after the tenth session because there was reason to believe that continuation was not likely to produce change.
>
> Worsened cases: treatment led to a worsening of the patient's condition.

Beyond defining and measuring efficacy, it is important to evaluate it in relation to the nature of the patient's problems. In other words, for a sound evaluation of the efficacy of a therapeutic model, one must make note of the type of problem the model confronts with greater or lesser efficacy (the efficacy differential).

The data presented hereunder are grouped into eight categories. The evaluation of efficacy, in addition to being applied to the entire sample, was also differentiated in regard to the types of problems treated. The definition — at times ambiguous — of the problem or disorder was made through consideration of the patient's prevalent or dominant symptoms. The classifications are as follows:

> Phobias
> Obsessive-compulsive disorders
> Sexual problems

Marital problems
Identity and relationship problems
Depressive disorders
Eating disorders
Psychoses or supposed psychoses

This empirically based set of categories is in keeping with the DSM III classifications of psychological and psychiatric diagnostic standards for all disorders except for marital problems, which — perhaps because they are purely relationship problems — are not included in these manuals.

It is important, nevertheless, to remember that the systemic and strategic approach avoids the traditional nosological and psychiatric classifications, insofar as they hardly take into account the complexity of human systems. We prefer to speak of problem typologies and their solutions. The classification presented here, apparently contradicting these traditional epistemological positions, was chosen with a view toward establishing a frame of reference that is not strictly limited to the systemic approach. We believe that this is the only way of allowing comparisons between the results of this therapeutic model and others.

This subdivision of problem typologies, based on the cases treated from January 1987 to September 1988 at the Strategic Therapy Center of Arezzo, cannot be considered a balanced case study. For some problem categories the number of cases treated is sufficiently representative, while for other disorders the number of treated cases is considerably less; therefore, a complete and reliable statistical evaluation of the differential efficacy of our model is not possible. Nevertheless, this does not eliminate the possibility of deducing interesting and useful information even from this breakdown (see Table 7.1).

One rarely examined aspect of therapy is its effectiveness (Garfield 1980), or its cost/benefit ratio. And yet, this aspect has great theoretical and social importance; in fact, there is quite a significant cost difference between the solution of a problem in three months and a solution in three years. The difference is in the cost, and above all in the fact that a person is going

Table 7.1. Treatment Efficacy:
Outcomes One Year After Last Session.

Type of Problem	Resolved		Considerably Improved		Little Improved		Unchanged		Worsened		Total Treated Cases	
	N	%	N	%	N	%	N	%	N	%	N	%
Phobia	32	78	7	17	2	5	-	-	-	-	41	100
Obsessive-compulsive	17	71	-	-	6	25	1	4	-	-	24	100
Sexual	10	67	2	13	5	20	-	-	-	-	15	100
Marital	9	100	-	-	-	-	-	-	-	-	9	100
Identity	8	57	3	21	3	21	-	-	-	-	14	100
Depressive	8	80	-	-	2	20	-	-	-	-	10	100
Eating	4	67	-	-	1	17	1	17	-	-	6	100
Psychoses or supposed psychoses	2	15	7	54	2	15	2	15	-	-	13	100
Total	90	69	19	14	21	14	4	3	-	-	134	100

to live better and more happily as soon as the problems that led him to therapy are solved. But oddly enough, as Garfield (1980) notes, what would seem to be a fundamental rule of professional ethics — the speedy solution of problems and suffering — has not been much considered by psychotherapists. Garfield explains this apparently incomprehensible attitude with the fact that for decades psychotherapeutic thought has been dominated by the idea that, to be effective, therapy must be prolonged, deep, and complex.

This view, typical of traditional psychotherapeutic theories, has been decisively refuted by the research on the comparative efficacy of psychotherapy. In fact, the data clearly demonstrate that there are no significant differences between results obtained in long-term therapy and those obtained in shorter therapy (Avnet, 1965; Muench, 1965; Schlien, 1957; Luborsky, Singer, and Luborsky, 1975; Garfield, Prager, and Bergin, 1971; Butcher and Koss, 1978; Harris, Kalis, and Freeman, 1963, 1964; Phillips and Wiener, 1966; Gurman and Kniskern, 1978). In some cases, the research even indicated that shorter-term therapy was more effective. The aforementioned lack of attention regarding these findings would then appear to be a consequence of resistance on the part of traditional psychotherapists to changing their theoretical convictions.

It would thus appear that for these therapists it is more important to save their sacred theories than to quickly and effectively help their patients.

Careful consideration of effectiveness should be an important factor in the analysis and evaluation of the power of a therapeutic model. The amount of time committed to obtaining a result qualifies the result itself; in fact, the relation between therapy's costs and benefits will be more positive the less prolonged the treatment.

Results

To measure the effectiveness of our work, we utilized a breakdown similar to that used to present efficacy (see Table 7.2).

Table 7.2. Duration of Treatment.

Type of Problem	Cases (N)	Median Duration (Sessions)	Minimum Duration (Sessions)	Maximum Duration (Sessions)
Phobia	41	15.6	6	34
Obsessive-compulsive	24	16.1	7	31
Sexual	15	12.0	5	42
Marital	9	16.4	5	34
Identity	14	13.1	5	33
Depressive	10	17.6	6	40
Eating	6	14.0	7	21
Psychoses or supposed psychoses	13	22.6	10	43
Total	132	15.9	6.4	34.8

Effectiveness was measured in terms of the median duration of treatment, both at the general level and at the differential level by type of disorder. In addition, effectiveness was judged by setting aside from the total sample all cases with positive outcome: the completely resolved cases and those considerably improved (see Table 7.3).

Table 7.3. Effectiveness of Treatment: Median Duration of Treatment for Resolved or Considerably Improved Cases.

Type of Problem	Resolved Cases		Considerably Improved Cases		Total Cases	
	N	Median Duration (Sessions)	N	Median Duration (Sessions)	N	Median Duration (Sessions)
Phobia	32	14.3	7	18.2	39	16.2
Obsessive-compulsive	17	12.5	-	-	17	12.5
Sexual	10	14.2	2	13.0	12	13.6
Marital	9	16.4	-	-	9	16.4
Identity	8	10.8	3	20.3	11	15.5
Depressive	8	18.7	-	-	8	18.7
Eating	4	13.7	-	-	4	13.7
Psychoses or supposed psychoses	2	42.0	7	21.8	9	31.9
Total	90	17.8	19	18.3	109	17.8

Final Considerations on the Results

Evaluation of our results leads us to several conclusions, about both the capacity of this specific interventive model and general themes of therapy evaluation.

The Sample

The sample comprises all cases treated at the Strategic Therapy Center of Arezzo from January 1987 to September 1988. Since the center is a private enterprise, the patients came for treatment of their own accord, and in that sense they represent a random sample. The only variables that all patients share are the request for therapy at the same center and the fact of being treated with strategic therapy.

The sample comprises 132 cases, although 149 persons had originally requested therapy (17 [11 percent] of them abandoned therapy during the first three sessions and were considered dropouts). The sample includes 53 men and 79 women, with a median age of twenty-six, the youngest being eight and the oldest seventy-one. The social standing and professional activities of the patients are quite disparate and heterogeneous. The only common element is that all patients were in a position to pay for the services of a private therapy center; none of them was in serious economic difficulty.

General Success

The efficacy of this type of treatment is clearly demonstrated in its high general success rate. The positive outcomes of treatment are 83 percent of the treated cases. In addition, this efficacy is even more evident in regard to specific problems, such as phobic disorders (agoraphobia and panic attacks), where there is a success rate of 95 percent. If we compare these data with the results of the research literature on the efficacy of different psychotherapeutic approaches (Andrews and Harvey, 1981; Bergin and Strupp, 1972; Garfield, 1981; Giles, 1983; Luborsky, Singer, and Luborsky, 1975; Sirigatti, 1988; Strupp and Hadley, 1979),

which estimate the positive success rate of various therapies —
according to the various approaches and research data — at 50
percent to 80 percent, it is obvious that the strategic approach
has an efficacy superior to the median. It also passed the follow-
up test one year after the end of therapy.

Success Over Time

The treatment efficacy of the strategic approach is maintained
over time. The percentage of relapses is quite low, and the results
obtained at the end of therapy are maintained in the majority
of cases through the third follow-up — after one year — making
future relapses or the emergence of substitute symptoms rather
unlikely. In accord with Garfield (1980), this refutes the sup-
position, common among therapists, that short-term therapies
are superficial and lead inevitably to relapses into the original
problem (or symptom displacement).

Treatment Effectiveness

Treatment effectiveness is the characteristic that, we believe,
distinguishes the results of strategic therapy from those of other
approaches. There is obviously quite a difference between therapy that lasts (on average) 14 sessions and one that lasts 835
(the average duration of psychoanalytic treatments in the Men-
ninger Foundation Psychotherapy Research Project, as reported
by Garfield, 1981). The real cost of the longer or shorter duration of therapy is not, it seems to us, primarily economic, but
has a bearing on the patient's quality of life. The difference between the successful treatment of a severely agoraphobic patient
in 14 sessions (three or four months) or in 150 sessions (three
or four years) is that in the former the patient feels considerably better after only a few months, whereas in the latter the
patient must continue to live for quite a long time dominated
by this problem. Referring again to Garfield (1980), it seems
crucial to establish which therapy will best serve a given patient's needs with the least expense, either economic or existential. Therapy must begin with these concerns in mind, but if

these procedures are not working or prove to be inadequate, it is then legitimate to move on to other procedures, which might prove to be more effective. Of course, not all human problems can be solved in a brief time, but, to be sure, one must try.

Once a specific form of therapy has shown its efficacy, its effectiveness becomes a factor of major consideration. If it is necessary to use "manipulative" strategies or "beneficial confusion" — as in many of the cases described in this book — we maintain that such tactics are most correct and ethical insofar as the goal is to help the patients solve their problems as quickly as possible. Therefore, "manipulation" and "beneficial confusion" are not instruments of torture, but strategies to break down patients' resistance to change, and thus lead to their feeling better with the least existential and economic costs.

References

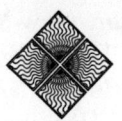

Alexander, F. *Psychoanalysis and Psychotherapy.* New York: Norton, 1956.

Alexander, F., and French, T. *Psychoanalytic Therapy.* New York: Ronald Press, 1946.

Andrews, G., and Harvey, R. "Does Psychotherapy Benefit Neurotic Patients? A Reanalysis of the Smith, Glass, and Miller Data." *Archives of General Psychiatry,* 1981, *38,* 1203–1208.

Ashby, W. R. *Design for a Brain.* New York: Wiley, 1954.

Ashby, W. R. *An Introduction to Cybernetics.* London: Methuen, 1956.

Austin, J. L. *How to Do Things with Words.* Cambridge, Mass.: Harvard University Press, 1962.

Avnet, H. H. "How Effective Is Short-Term Therapy?" In L. R. Wolberg (ed.), *Short-Term Psychotherapy.* New York: Grune and Stratton, 1965.

Balint, M. *The Basic Fault.* London: Tavistock, 1968.

Bandler, R., and Grinder, J. *Patterns of the Hypnotic Technique of Milton H. Erickson, M.D.* Palo Alto, Calif.: Meta Publications, 1975a.

Bandler, R., and Grinder, J. *The Structure of Magic.* Palo Alto, Calif.: Meta Publications, 1975b.

Bannister, D., and Fransella, F. *Inquiring Man: The Theory of Personal Constructs.* Harmondsworth, England: Penguin, 1977.

Bateson, G. "Cybernetic Explanation." *American Behavioral Scientist,* 1967, *10,* 29–32.

Bateson, G. *Steps to an Ecology of Mind.* New York: Ballantine, 1972.

Bateson, G. *Mind and Nature.* New York: Bantam Books, 1979.

Bateson, G., and Jackson, D. D. "Some Varieties of Pathogenic Organization." In *Disorders of Communication* (Research Publications, Association for Research in Nervous and Mental Disease), 1964, *42,* 270–283.

Bateson, G., Jackson, D. D., Haley, J., and Weakland, J. H. "Toward a Theory of Schizophrenia." *Behavioral Sciences,* 1956, *1,* 251–264.

Bergin, A. E., and Strupp, H. H. *Changing Frontiers in the Science of Psychotherapy.* Chicago: Aldine, 1972.

Bergman, J. S. *Fishing for Barracuda: Pragmatics of Brief Systemic Therapy.* New York: Norton, 1985.

Bloch, S. *To Be a Therapist: The Teaching and Learning.* New York: Brunner/Mazel, 1984.

Brown, G. S. *Laws of Form.* New York: Bantam, 1973.

Butcher, J. N., and Koss, M. P. *M.M.P.I. Research on Brief and Crisis-Oriented Therapies.* In S. L. Garfield and A. E. Bergin (eds.), *Handbook of Psychotherapy and Behavior Change.* (2nd ed.) New York: Wiley, 1978.

Cialdini, R. B. *How and Why People Agree to Things.* New York: William Morrow, 1984.

Dini, V. *Il potere delle antiche madri* (Maternal power in ancient times). Turin, Italy: Boringhieri, 1980.

Elster, J. *Ulysses and the Sirens.* Cambridge: Cambridge University Press, 1979.

Erickson, M. H., and Rossi, E. L. (eds.). *The Collected Papers of Milton H. Erickson on Hypnosis.* 4 vols. New York: Irvington, 1982.

Erickson, M. H., Rossi, E. L., and Rossi, S. I. *Hypnotic Realities: The Induction of Clinical Hypnosis and Forms of Indirect Suggestion.* New York: Irvington, 1979.

Fachinelli, E. *Claustrofilia.* Milan, Italy: Adelphi, 1983.

Fisch, R., Weakland, J. H., and Segal, L. *The Tactics of Change.* San Francisco: Jossey-Bass, 1982.

Foerster, H. von. "Thoughts and Notes on Cognition." In P. L. Garvin (ed.), *Cognition: A Multiple View.* New York: Plenum, 1970.

Foerster, H. von. "Kybernetik einer Erkenntnistheorie" (Cybernetic Epistemology). In W. D. Keidel, W. Handler, and M. Spring (eds.), *Kybernetik und Bionik* (Cybernetics and Bionics). Munich: Oldenburg, 1974.

Foerster, H. von. *Observing Systems.* Seaside, Calif.: Intersystems Publications, 1981.

Foerster, H. von. "On Constructing a Reality." In P. Watzlawick (ed.), *The Invented Reality.* New York: Norton, 1984.

Frankl, V. E. "Paradoxical Intention." *American Journal of Psychotherapy,* 1960, *14,* 520–535.

Freud, S. "New Introductory Lectures on Psycho-Analysis." In J. Strachey (ed. and trans.), *The Complete Psychological Works of Sigmund Freud.* Vol. 22. London: Hogarth Press, 1964.

Garfield, S. L. *Psychotherapy: An Eclectic Approach.* New York: Wiley, 1980.

Garfield, S. L. "Psychotherapy: A 40-Year Appraisal." *American Psychologist,* 1981, *2,* 174–183.

Garfield, S. L., Prager, R. A., and Bergin, A. E. "Evaluation of Outcome in Psychotherapy." *Journal of Consulting and Clinical Psychology,* 1971, *37,* 307–313.

Giannattasio, E., and Nencini, R. *Conoscenza e modellizzazione nella psicologia* (Knowledge and Model Building in Psychology). Rome: La Goliardica, 1983.

Giles, T. R. "Probable Superiority of Behavioral Interventions: I: Traditional Comparative Outcome." *Journal of Behavioral Therapy Experimental Psychiatry,* 1983, *14,* 29–32.

Glasersfeld, E. von. "Cybernetic Experience and Concept of Self." In M. N. Ozer (ed.), *A Cybernetic Approach to Assessment of Children: Towards More Humane Use of Human Beings.* Boulder, Colo.: Westview Press, 1979.

Glasersfeld, E. von. "An Introduction to Radical Constructivism." In P. Watzlawick (ed.), *The Invented Reality.* New York: Norton, 1984.

Glover, E. *Freud or Jung?* New York: Meridian Books, 1956.

Greenberg, G. "Problem-Focused Brief Family Interactional

Psychotherapy." In M. D. Wolberg, L. Marvin, and P. D. Aronson (eds.), *Group and Family Therapy*. New York: Brunner/Mazel, 1980.

Gurman, A. S., and Kniskern, D. P. "Research on Marital and Family Therapy." In S. Garfield and A. E. Bergin (eds.), *Handbook of Psychotherapy and Behavior Change*. (2nd ed.) New York: Wiley, 1978.

Haley, J. *Advanced Techniques of Hypnosis and Therapy: Selected Papers of Milton Erickson, M.D.* New York: Grune and Stratton, 1967.

Haley, J. *Uncommon Therapy: The Psychiatric Techniques of Milton Erickson, M.D.* New York: Norton, 1973.

Haley, J. *Problem-Solving Therapy*. San Francisco: Jossey-Bass, 1976.

Haley, J. *Conversations with Milton Erickson, M.D.* Vol. 1: *Changing Individuals*. Vol. 2: *Changing Couples*. Vol. 3: *Changing Families and Children*. Chicago: Triangle Press, 1985.

Harris, M. R., Kalis, B., and Freeman, E. "Precipitating Stress: An Approach to Brief Therapy." *American Journal of Psychotherapy*, 1963, *17*, 465–471.

Harris, M. R., Kalis, B., and Freeman, E. "An Approach to Short-Term Psychotherapy." *Mind*, 1964, *2*, 198–206.

Herr, J., and Weakland, J. H. *Counseling Elders and Their Families*. New York: Springer, 1979.

Hoffman, L. *Foundations of Family Therapy*. New York: Basic Books, 1981.

Hugo, V. *Les Misérables*. New York: American Publishers Corporation, n.d.

Jakobson, R. *Essais de linguistique générale* (Essays in General Linguistics). Paris: Editions de Minuit, 1963.

Kelly, G. A. *The Psychology of Personal Constructs*. (2 vols.) New York: Norton, 1955.

Kuhn, T. *The Structure of Scientific Revolutions*. Chicago: University of Chicago Press, 1970.

Lankton, S., and Lankton, C. H. *The Answer Within: A Clinical Framework of Ericksonian Hypnotherapy*. New York: Brunner/Mazel, 1983.

Luborsky, L., Singer, B., and Luborsky, L. "Comparative Studies of Psychotherapies: Is It True That Everyone Has

Won and All Must Have Prizes?" *Archives of General Psychiatry,* 1975, *132,* 995–1004.

Madanes, C. *Strategic Family Therapy.* San Francisco: Jossey-Bass, 1981.

Mally, E. *Grundgesetze des Sollens* (Basic Laws of Moral Obligations). Graz: Leuscher und Lubenky, 1926.

Maturana, H. R. "Biology of Language: The Epistemology of Reality." In G. A. Miller and E. Lennberg (eds.), *Psychology and Biology of Language and Thought.* New York: Academic Press, 1978.

Mayo, E. *The Human Problems of Industrial Civilization.* New York: Macmillan, 1933.

Montalvo, B., and Haley, J. "In Defense of Child Therapy." *Family Process,* 1973, *12,* 227–244.

Muench, G. A. "An Investigation of the Efficacy of Time-Limited Psychotherapy." *Journal of Counseling Psychology,* 1965, *12,* 294–299.

Nardone, G. (ed.). *Modelli di psicoterapia a confronto* (Confrontational Psychotherapy). Rome: IL Ventaglio, 1988.

Neumann, J. von, and Morgenstern, O. *Theory of Games and Economic Behavior.* Princeton, N.J.: Princeton University Press, 1944.

Phillips, D. "The Influence of Suggestion on Suicide: Substantive and Theoretical Implications of the Werther Effect." *American Sociological Review,* 1974, *39,* 340–354.

Phillips, D. "Suicide, Motor Vehicle Fatalities, and the Mass Media: Evidence Toward a Theory of Suggestion." *American Journal of Sociology,* 1979, *84,* 1150–1174.

Phillips, D. "Airplane Accident, Murder, and the Mass Media: Toward a Theory of Imitation and Suggestion." *Social Forces,* 1980, *58,* 1001–1024.

Phillips, E. L., and Wiener, D. N. *Short-Term Psychotherapy and Structural Behavior Change.* New York: McGraw-Hill, 1966.

Piaget, J. *The Construction of Reality in the Child.* New York: Basic Books, 1954. (Originally published 1937.)

Piaget, J. *Genetic Epistemology.* New York: Columbia University Press, 1970.

Piaget, J. *Biology and Knowledge.* Chicago: University of Chicago Press, 1971.

Popper, K. R. *Objective Knowledge.* London: Oxford University Press, 1972.

Popper, K. R. *Realism and the Aim of Science.* London: Hutchinson, 1983.

Prigogine, I. *From Being to Becoming.* San Francisco: Freeman, 1980.

Rabkin, R. *Strategic Psychotherapy.* New York: Basic Books, 1977.

Riedl, R. *Biologie der Erkenntis* (Biology of Cognition). Hamburg: Parey, 1980.

Ritterman, M. *Using Hypnosis in Family Therapy.* San Francisco: Jossey-Bass, 1983.

Rosen, S. "The Values and Philosophy of Milton Erickson." In J. Zeig (ed.), *Ericksonian Approaches to Hypnosis and Psychotherapy.* New York: Brunner/Mazel, 1982.

Rosenthal, R. *Experimenter Effects in Behavioral Research.* New York: Appleton-Century-Crofts, 1966.

Salzman, L. "Reply to Critics." *International Journal of Psychiatry,* 1968, *6,* 473–476.

Selvini-Palazzoli, M., Cirillo, S., Selvini, M., and Fiorentino, A. M. *Family Games.* New York: Norton, 1989.

Schimmel, A. (ed.). *Die orientalische Katze* (The Oriental Cat). Cologne: Diederichs, 1983.

Schlien, J. M. "Time-Limited Psychotherapy: An Experimental Investigation of Practical Values and Theoretical Implications." *Journal of Counseling Psychology,* 1957, *4,* 318–329.

Simon, B. F., Stierlin, H., and Wynne, C. L. *The Language of Family Therapy: A Systemic Vocabulary and Sourcebook.* New York: Family Process, 1985.

Sirigatti, S. "La ricerca valutativa in psicoterapia: modelli e prospettive" (Outcome Research in Psychotherapy: Models and Perspectives). In G. Nardone (ed.), *Modelli di psicoterapia a confronto* (Models of Confrontational Psychotherapy). Rome: Il Ventaglio, 1988.

Stolzenberg, G. *Can an Inquiry into the Foundations of Mathematics Tell Us Anything Interesting About Mind?* New York: Academic Press, 1978.

Strupp, H. H., and Hadley, S. W. "Specific Versus Nonspecific Factors in Psychotherapy: A Controlled Study of Outcome." *Archives of General Psychiatry,* 1979, *36,* 1125–1136.

Vaihinger, H. *The Philosophy of "As If."* (C. K. Ogden, trans.) New York: Harcourt Brace, 1924.

Varela, F. "A Calculus for Self-Reference." *International Journal of General Systems,* 1975, *2,* 5–24.

Varela, F. *Principles of Biological Autonomy.* New York: North Holland, 1979.

Watzlawick, P. *How Real Is Real?* New York: Random House, 1976.

Watzlawick, P. *The Language of Change.* New York: Basic Books, 1978.

Watzlawick, P. (ed.). *The Invented Reality.* New York: Norton, 1984.

Watzlawick, P. "Hypnotherapy Without Trance." In J. Zeig, (ed.), *Ericksonian Psychotherapy.* Vol. 1: *Structure.* New York: Brunner/Mazel, 1985.

Watzlawick, P., Beavin, J., and Jackson, D. D. *Pragmatics of Human Communication: A Study on Interactional Patterns, Pathologies and Paradoxes.* New York: Norton, 1967.

Watzlawick, P., and Weakland, J. H. (eds.). *The Interactional View.* New York: Norton, 1977.

Watzlawick, P., Weakland, J. H., and Fisch, R. *Change: Principles of Problem Formation and Problem Solution.* New York: Norton, 1974.

Weakland, J. H., Fisch, R., Watzlawick, P., and Bodin, A. "Brief Therapy: Focused Problem Resolution." *Family Process,* 1974, *13,* 141–168.

Whitehead, A. N., and Russell, B. *Principia Mathematica.* 3 vols. Cambridge: Cambridge University Press, 1910–1913.

Wiener, N. "Time, Communications, and the Nervous System." In R. W. Miner (ed.), *Teleological Mechanisms* (Annals of the New York Academy of Sciences), *50* (art. 4), 1947.

Zeig, J. *A Teaching Seminar with Milton H. Erickson.* New York: Brunner/Mazel, 1980.

Zeig, J. *Ericksonian Psychotherapy.* New York: Brunner/Mazel, 1985.

Zeig, J. (ed.). *The Evolution of Psychotherapy.* New York: Brunner/Mazel, 1987.

Recommended Readings

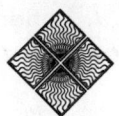

Bergin, A. E., and Lambert, M. J. "The Evaluation of Therapeutic Outcomes." In S. L. Garfield and A. E. Bergin (eds.), *Handbook of Psychotherapy and Behavior Change.* (2nd ed.) New York: Wiley, 1978.

Bodin, A. "The Interactional View: Family Therapy Approaches of the Mental Research Institute." In A. S. Gurman and D. P. Kniskern (eds.), *The Handbook of Family Therapy.* New York: Brunner/Mazel, 1980.

Chambers, G. S., and Hamlin, R. "The Validity of Judgments Based on 'Blind' Rorschach Records." *Journal of Consulting Psychology,* 1957, *21,* 105–109.

Fiora, E., Pedrabissi, I., and Salvini, A. *Pluralismo teorico e pragmatismo conoscitivo in psicologia della personalità* (Theoretical Pluralism and Cognitive Pragmatism in the Psychology of Personality). Milan: Giuffrè, 1988.

Fisch, R., Weakland, J. H., Watzlawick, P., Segal, L., Hoebel, F., and Deardorf, M. *Learning Brief Therapy: An Introductory Training Manual.* Palo Alto, Calif.: Mental Research Institute, 1975.

Fisch, R., Watzlawick, P., Weakland, J. H., and Bodin, A. "On Unbecoming Family Therapists." In A. Ferber, M. Mendelson, and A. Napier (eds.), *The Book of Family Therapy.* New York: Science House, 1982.

Frank, J. D. "Therapeutic Components of Psychotherapy: A
   Twenty-five Year Progress Report of Research." *Journal of
   Consulting and Clinical Psychology,* 1971, *37,* 307–313.

Gödel, K. *On Formally Undecidable Propositions of Principia Mathematica and Related Systems, I.* London: Oliver and Boyd, 1962.

Kant, I. *Critica della ragion pura* (Critique of pure reason). Bari:
   Laterza, 1985.

Lewis, J. M. *To Be a Therapist: The Teaching and Learning.* New
   York: Brunner/Mazel, 1978.

Liddle, H. A. "Diagnosis and Assessment in Family Therapy:
   A Comparative Analysis of Six Schools of Thought." In B.
   Keeney (ed.), *Diagnosis and Assessment in Family Therapy.* Rock-
   ville, Md.: Aspen Publications, 1982.

Maisondieu, J., and Matayer, L. *Les thérapies familiales* (The
   Family Therapies). Paris: Press Universitaires de France,
   1986.

Minguzzi, G. F. "È possibile valutare i risultati della psicoterapia?" (Can the Results of Psychotherapy Be Evaluated?). *Il
   giornale italiano de psicologia* (The Italian Journal of Psychology), 1986, *13* (1), 7–13.

Nietzsche, F. *La gaia scienza* (The Gay Science). Milan: Adelphi, 1965.

Rhodes, R. *Hypnosis: Theory, Practice, and Application.* New York:
   Citadel Press, 1965.

Selvini-Palazzoli, M., Boscolo, L., Cecchin, G., and Prata, G.
   Paradox and Counterparadox. New York: Jason Aronson, 1978.

Segal, L. "Focused Problem Resolution." In E. Tolsen and W. J.
   Reid (eds.), *Models of Family Therapy.* New York: Columbia
   University Press, 1980.

Sirigatti, S. "Behavior Therapy and Therapist Variables: A-B
   Distinction in the Treatment of Monophobias." *Bollettino di
   psicologia applicata* (Bulletin of Applied Psychology), 1975, pp.
   127–129.

Sluzki, C. E., and Donald, C. R. *Double Bind: The Foundation
   of the Communicational Approach to the Family.* New York: Grune
   and Stratton, 1979.

Smith, M. L., Glass, G. U., and Miller, T. I. *The Benefit of
   Psychotherapy.* Baltimore: Johns Hopkins University Press,
   1980.

Smith, M. L., Glass, G. U., and Miller, T. I. *The Benefit of Psychotherapy.* Baltimore: Johns Hopkins University Press, 1980.

Varela, F. "The Creative Circle." In P. Watzlawick (ed.), *The Invented Reality.* New York: Norton, 1988.

Vico, G. *De antiquissima italorum sapientia* (The Wisdom of the Ancient Italics). Naples: Stamperia de' Classici Latini, 1958.

Wester, W. C., and Smith, H. A. *Clinical Hypnosis.* Philadelphia: Lippincott, 1984.

Wiener, N. *The Human Use of Human Beings: Cybernetics and Society.* (2nd ed.) New York: Avon, 1967.

Wiener, N. *Cybernetics, or Control and Communication in the Animal and the Machine.* (2nd ed.) Cambridge, Mass.: MIT Press, 1975.

Index

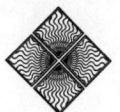